EPIDURAL ANALGESIA – CURRENT VIEWS AND APPROACHES

Edited by **Sotonye Fyneface-Ogan**

Epidural Analgesia – Current Views and Approaches
Edited by Sotonye Fyneface-Ogan

Published by InTech
Janeza Trdine 9, 51000 Rijeka, Croatia

Publishing Process Manager Ivona Lovric

Technical Editor Teodora Smiljanic

Cover Designer InTech Design Team

Additional hard copies can be obtained from orders@intechopen.com

Epidural Analgesia – Current Views and Approaches, Edited by Sotonye Fyneface-Ogan
p. cm.
ISBN 978-953-51-0332-5

For EU product safety concerns:
IN TECH d.o.o., Prolaz Marije Krucifikse Kozulić 3, 51000 Rijeka, Croatia,
info@intechopen.com or visit our website at intechopen.com.

Meet the editor

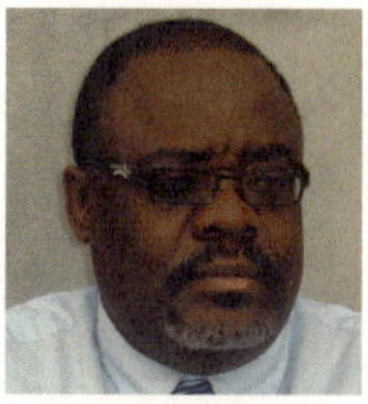

Dr Sotonye Fyneface-Ogan, FWACS attended medical school at the College of Health Sciences, University of Port Harcourt, Port Harcourt, Nigeria, and graduated in 1989. He is a Senior Lecturer in Anesthesiology and a Fellow of the West African College of Surgeons (WACS). His post-fellowship training in Obstetric Anesthesiology was at the Edith Wolfson Medical Centre, Holon, Israel. He is the President of the League of Obstetric Anesthesiologists of Nigeria (LOAN) and is one of the pioneers and leaders in the field of obstetric analgesia in Nigeria. He has many scientific papers to his name and is a reviewer of many medical journals.

Contents

Preface

The World Health Organization defines pain as "an unpleasant sensory or emotional experience associated with actual or potential tissue damage, or described in terms of such damage". According to Baszanger, "[p]ain is a person's private experience, to which no one else has direct access and cannot be reduced by objectification, it cannot, ultimately, be stabilized as an unquestionable fact that can serve as the basis of medical practice and thus organize relations between professional and lay persons". Therefore pain, whatever the source, must be treated. Epidural analgesia has been extensively used to relieve pain of some regions of the human body.

Epidural analgesia is now frequently used to carry out postoperative and labor analgesia. First described in 1901 by Corning, the exploration of the epidural space is technically demanding and requires a good knowledge of the relevant anatomy and contents of the space.

The use of this space for various purposes in obstetrics has improved over the years. One publication by the American Society of Anesthesiologists Task Force on Obstetric Anesthesia illustrates consistent improvement of knowledge in this area. Epidural analgesia is produced with the use of low dose local anesthetics (such as bupivacaine, ropivacaine, lidocaine, levobupivacaine), opioids, or alpha agonists alone, or in combination. It is known to provide superior regional analgesia over conventional systemic routes (intravenous or enteral), with minimal systemic side effects (nausea, sedation, constipation). In low doses these local anesthetics produce more sensory block and with less motor block. However the aim of striking a difficult balance between the lowest motor block possible (to facilitate labour and vaginal delivery, and even allow ambulation) and an optimal analgesia could be a challenging one. Local anesthetic concentrations as low as 0.0625% bupivacaine have been used with fentanyl 20 micrograms for epidural analgesia for labor.

Generally speaking, agents injected into the epidural space are distributed by three main pathways: diffusion through the dura into the cerebrospinal fluid (CSF), then to the spinal cord or nerve roots; vascular uptake by the vessels in the epidural space into systemic circulation; and uptake by the fat in the epidural space, creating a drug depot from which the drug can eventually enter the CSF or the systemic circulation.

Epidural analgesia is a commonly employed technique of providing pain relief during labor. The number of parturients given intrapartum epidural analgesia is reported to be over 50% at many institutions in the United States and United Kingdom. While this figure is much lower in some developed countries, intrapartum epidural analgesia is almost non-existent in many parts of low resource countries as a result of the dearth of manpower and equipment. A survey of obstetric anesthesia in the United States indicated that the percentage of women given intrapartum epidural analgesia increased from 22% in 1981 to 51% in 1992 at hospitals performing at least 1,500 deliveries annually. The increased availability of epidural analgesia and the favorable experiences of women who have had painless labor with epidural block have reshaped the expectations of pregnant women entering labor.

Although epidural analgesia is the most widely used method of pain relief in childbirth it does not mean that the method is free of complications or contraindications, but these are considered to be of minor importance and a generally infrequent event. In general, the gains outweigh the losses and epidurals are now regarded as a safe method for both mothers and babies.

Pain from labor or otherwise does not involve only the patient, or the expectant mother, but their families and relations as well as the professionals who assist the patient and who give sense and meaning to the pain of others through compassion, acknowledgement and admiration; sentiments that the sufferer perceives and analyses as part of the meaning of such suffering, and which finally legitimizes it or not, gives it meaning or not, and therefore makes it seem "useful" or not. Pain must be relieved no matter the gender or the age!

Epidural analgesia has been well-known to confer excellent pain relief and complete dynamic analgesia leading to a substantial reduction in the surgical stress response. It provides favorable effects on coagulation and homeostasis, as well as on cardiorespiratory, gastrointestinal and immune functions, all these potential positive influences being theoretically translated into an improved quality of patient recovery.

Epidural analgesia can be administered by intermittent boluses (by a clinician or by patient controlled epidural analgesia (PCEA) using an appropriate pump); continuous infusion; or a combination thereof. PCEA is used to supplement a basal rate, to allow a patient to manage breakthrough pain in order to meet their individual analgesic requirements. Like Intravenous Patient Controlled Analgesia (IV PCA), PCEA can provide more timely pain relief, more control for the patient, and convenience for both the patient and nurse to reduce the time required to obtain and administer required supplemental boluses. Unlike IV PCA, the lockout interval of PCEA varies widely based on the lipid solubility of the opioid administered, from 10 minutes with fentanyl to 60 to 90 minutes when morphine is used. If local anesthetic is used, the lockout interval is taught to be at least 15 minutes to allow for peak effect of the supplemental local anesthetic dose.

Epidural analgesia has been found to be very useful for postoperative pain relief in paediatric patients. Some of the numerous benefits include earlier ambulation, rapid weaning from ventilators, reduced time spent in a catabolic state, and lowered circulating stress hormone levels. Specific protocols and guidelines tailored to suit the pediatric patients can increase the success of placement, optimize the efficacy of analgesia and increase overall safety. These specific epidural protocols are directed at how to confirm correct catheter placement, which type of age-specific infusion to use and how much is safe, and how to treat side effects. Epidural analgesia is useful as part of a multimodal approach to acute and chronic pain management in children. The single S+ isomers, ropivacaine and levobupivacaine, are the drugs of choice in pediatric practice. The reduced cardiac and central nervous system toxicity, and less motor blockade, suggest that these agents may be more beneficial, particularly in infants and neonates. The maximum suggested dosage for racemic bupivacaine (0.2mg/kg/h for infants and neonates, 0.4 mg/kg/ h for older children) has led to improved safety of continuous epidural infusions.

The administration of pharmacologic active agents to geriatric patients is complicated by the adverse conditions imposed by the aging process such as diminished functional activity, decreased metabolic rate, decreased function of liver and kidneys, increased sensitivity to anoxia and loss of blood, and increased drug sensitivity is likewise increasing in importance. Epidural analgesia has been found to reduce the intravenous opioid requirements in the geriatric population following surgeries of thoracic, upper abdominal, lower abdominal region.

Generally, epidural analgesia is time-consuming; it requires specific technical skills, pharmacological abilities and professional surveillance. Clearly, epidural analgesia is not devoid of risks and failures may occur.

Sotonye Fyneface-Ogan B.Med.Sc, M.B;B.S, PgDA, FWACS
Senior Lecturer
Head of Department of Anesthesiology
Faculty of Clinical Sciences
College of Health Sciences
University of Port Harcourt,
Port Harcourt,
Nigeria

1

Anatomy and Clinical Importance of the Epidural Space

Sotonye Fyneface-Ogan
Department of Anaesthesiology, Faculty of Clinical Sciences, College of Health Sciences, University of Port Harcourt, Nigeria

1. Introduction

The epidural space is one of the most explored spaces of the human body. This exploration demands a good knowledge of the relevant anatomy and contents of the space. First described in 1901 (Corning JL, 1901), the epidural space is an anatomic compartment between the dural sheath and the spinal canal. In some areas it is a real space and in others only a potential space.

Various methods have been used to study the anatomy of the epidural space by investigators. Methods such as epiduroscopy in cadavers and patients, anatomical dissection, Magnetic Resonance Imaging (MRI), Computerized Tomographic epidurography (Yan et al., 2010), epidural injections of resins and the use of cryomicrotome sectioning in cadavers frozen soon after death (Hogan QH, 1991), have been used to demonstrate the inner layout of the space.

The use of the term 'space' has been controversial amongst anatomists. It is argued that the term would be more appropriate for the subarachnoid space than the epidural. It is claimed that the epidural space is not an open anatomical space whether in life or death. The only time a space is present is when the dura mater is artificially separated from the overlying vertebral canal by injection of contrast media or solutions of local anesthetics (Parkin & Harrison, 1985).

2. Embryology of the epidural space

Histological transverse sections of human lumbar spines of adults and fetuses aged 13, 15, 21, 32 and 39 weeks (menstrual age) were studied (Hamid et al., 2002). It was found that at the 13th week the epidural space had been filled with connective tissue and the dura mater was attached to the posterior longitudinal ligament. By the 13th week of embryonic development, three distinct stages had been formed and differentiate progressively within the connective tissue (Rodionov et al., 2010).

These are:

- the primary epidural space (embryos of 16-31 mm crown-rump length (CRL));
- reduction of the primary epidural space (embryos of 35-55 mm CRL);

- the secondary epidural space (embryos of 60-70 mm CRL and fetuses of 80-90 mm CRL).

It has been found that the morphogenesis of the primary epidural space is determined by the formative influence of the spinal cord and its dura mater, while that of the secondary epidural space is determined by the walls of the vertebral canal (Rodionov et al., 2010).

Within this period of embryonic life, the posterior longitudinal ligament (PLL) attaches to the vertebral body beside the midline, and to the posterior edge of intervertebral disc. The anterior internal vertebral venous plexus is formed and located anterolaterally and anteromedially. At 15 weeks, the posterior longitudinal ligament develops better into deep and superficial layers. At 21 weeks, the attachment between the dura mater and PLL was ligament-like at the level of the vertebral body (Hamid et al., 2002). At 32 weeks, the dura mater was adherent to the superficial layer of PLL. At 39 weeks, groups of adipocytes begin to develop.

3. Anatomy

The vertebral column is made up of 24 individual vertebrae comprising 7 cervical, 12 thoracic and 5 lumbar while 5 sacral vertebrae are fused and the 3-5 coccygeal bones, though fused, remain rudimentary. These vertebrae house the epidural and the subarachnoid spaces.

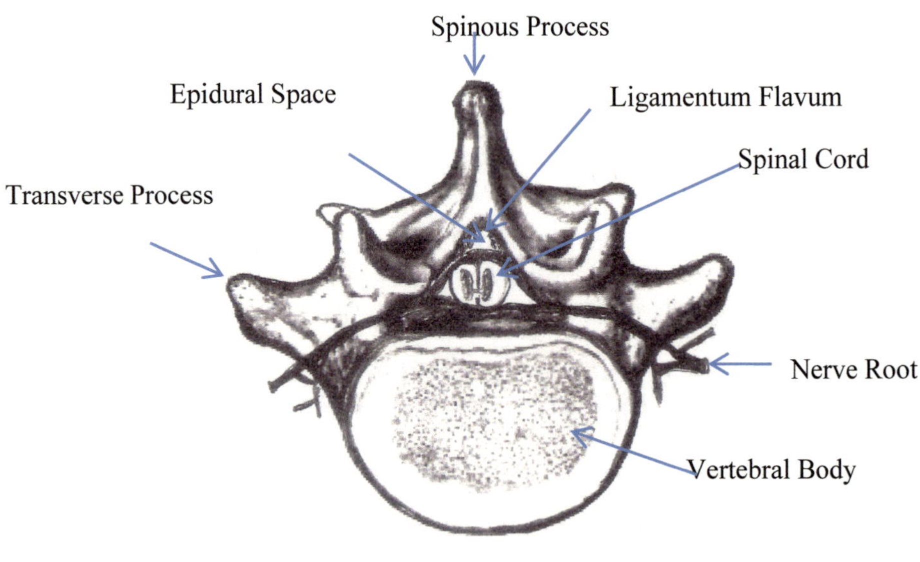

Transverse Section of the Lumbar Vertebra

3.1 Measurement of the epidural space

The epidural space is most roomy at the upper thoracic levels. The epidural space at the posterior space in the adult measures about 0.4 mm at C7-T1, 7.5 mm in the upper thoracic region, 4.1 mm at T11-12 region and 4-7 mm in the lumbar region, (Nickallis & Kokri, 1986). The space is far greater than that of the subarachnoid space at the same level. It takes about

1.5 - 2.0 ml of a local anesthetic to block a spinal segment in the epidural space while the volume (0.3 ml) is far less in the subarachnoid space for a similar block. It has been shown (Macintosh and Lee, 1973) that the paravertebral spaces, both serially and contralaterally, communicate with each other in the epidural space.

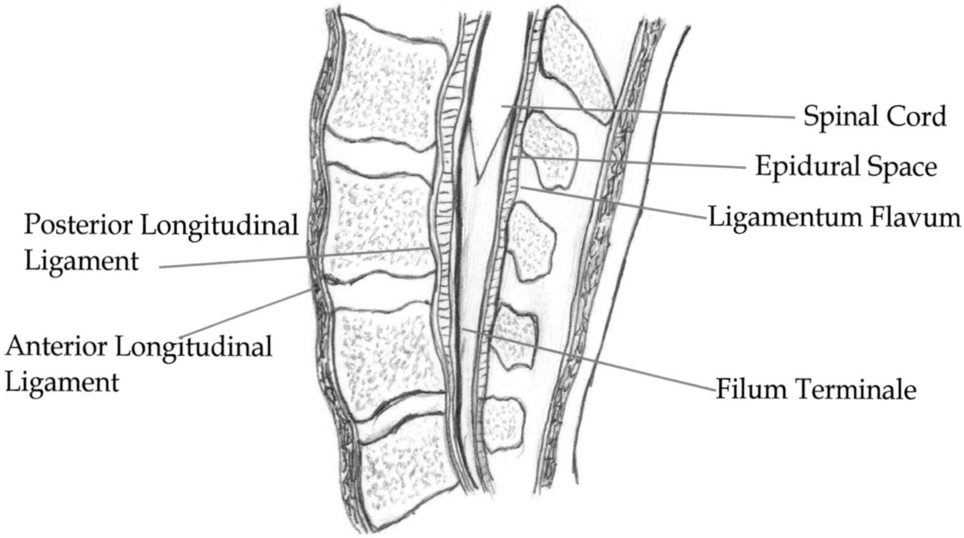

Sagittal section of the Lumbar Region

3.2 Shape and size of the epidural space

These are largely determined by the shape of the lumbar vertebral canal and the position and size of the dural sac within it. It has been suggested that though merely a potential space (Bromage, 1978) it could be up to 5 mm in depth (Husemeyer & White, 1980).

3.3 Types of epidural space

The epidural space can be categorized into cervical, thoracic, lumbar and sacral epidural spaces. These spaces can be defined according to their margins. At the cervical epidural space, there is a fusion of the spinal and periosteal layers of dura mater at the foramen magnum to lower margin of the 7th cervical vertebra. While the thoracic epidural space is formed by the lower margin of C7 to the upper margin of L1, the lumbar epidural space is formed by the lower margin of L1 vertebra to the upper margin of S1 vertebra. The sacral epidural space is formed by the upper margin of S1 to sacrococcygeal membrane.

3.4 Boundaries of the epidural space

The epidural space is bounded superiorly by the fusion of the spinal and periosteal layers of the dura mater at the foramen magnum. Inferiorly, it is bound by the sacrococcygeal membrane. The space is bounded anteriorly by the posterior longitudinal ligament, vertebral bodies and discs while the pedicles and intervertebral foraminae form the lateral boundary. The ligamentum flavum, capsule of facet joints and the laminae form the posterior boundary of the epidural space.

3.5 Pressure of the epidural space

The epidural space with the exception of the sacral region is said to be under negative pressure. The significance of the negative pressure has been a point of considerable argument. It has been hypothesized that the initial or 'true' negative pressure encountered when a needle first enters the epidural space could be due to initial bulging of the ligamentum flavum in front of the advancing needle followed by its rapid return to the resting position once the needle has perforated the ligament. The bulging has been confirmed to occur in fresh cadavers, and pressure studies carried out during performance of epidural blocks in patients lend weight to this hypothesis (Zarzur E, 1984).

Negative pressure can be magnified by increasing and reduced by decreasing the flexion of the spine. The negative pressure appears to be positive when the vertebral column is straightened. Depending on the position of the needle, two different components of negative pressure have been recognized. A basal value ranging from -1 to -7 cmH_2O could be observed when entering the epidural space. It remains stable providing the patient is well relaxed. An artefactual component up to -30 cmH_2O could appear if needle is further advanced against the dural sac (Usubiaja et al., 1967).

The epidural space identification is frequently dependent on the negative pressure within this space. It has been demonstrated that the epidural pressure is more negative in the sitting position than in the lateral decubitus position especially in the thoracic region. It therefore suggests that the space is better identified in the sitting position when the hanging drop technique is used to identify the epidural space (Gil et al., 2008).

3.6 The contents of the epidural space

This space contains semi-liquid fat, lymphatics, arteries, loose areolar connective tissue, the spinal nerve roots, and extensive plexus of veins. The epidural contents are contained in a series of circumferentially discontinuous compartments separated by zones where the dura contacts the wall of the vertebral canal (Hogan, 1998).

3.6.1 Fat

The distribution of the epidural fat has been studied. It is now known that the epidural space contains abundant epidural fat that distributes along the spinal canal in a predictable pattern (Reina et al., 2006). Fat cells are also abundant in the dura that forms the sleeves around spinal nerve roots but they are not embedded within the laminas that form the dura mater of the dural sac. The fat in the epidural space buffers the pulsatile movements of the dural sac and protects nerve structure, creates a reservoir of lipophilic substances, and facilitates the movement of the dural sac over the periosteum of the spinal column during flexion and extension. The epidural fat has a continuous pattern of distribution that assumes a metameric pattern especially in the adult human (Reina et al., 2006). Drugs stored in fat, inside dural sleeves, could have a greater impact on nerve roots than drugs stored in epidural fat, given that the concentration of fat is proportionally higher inside nerve root sleeves than in the epidural space, and that the distance between nerves and fat is shorter.

Similarly, changes in fat content and distribution caused by different pathologies may alter the absorption and distribution of drugs injected in the epidural space (Reina et al., 2009).

The fat is largely distributed along the dorsal margin of the space, where it assumes triangular capsular shapes and linked to the midline of the ligamentum flavum by a vascular pedicle. The clinical significance of the fat distribution is related to the pharmacokinetics of drugs including local anesthetics injected into the space leaving a minute quantity of the agent to react with the nerve roots, and the slight resistance experienced during the insertion of an epidural catheter.

3.6.2 Lymphatics

The lymphatics of the epidural space are concentrated in the region of the dural roots where they remove foreign materials including microorganisms from the subarachnoid and epidural spaces.

3.6.3 Vertebral venous plexus

The internal vertebral venous plexus has been extensively studied and found to be located in the epidural space (Domisse, 1975; Parkin and Harrison, 1985; Brockstein et al., 1994). This plexus of veins is thought to be frequently involved in a bloody or traumatic tap (Mehl, 1986) during needle placement in the epidural space. The internal vertebral venous plexus consists of four interconnecting longitudinal vessels, two anterior and two posterior. The external vertebral plexus (EVP) in contrast, lies peripheral to the vertebrae and is made of the anterior and posterior external vertebral plexuses (Williams et al., 1989). The EVP is situated anterior to the vertebral bodies and in relation to the laminae, spinous processes, transverse processes and articular processes respectively.

These veins communicate with the segmental veins of the neck, the intercostal, azygos and lumbar veins. With the veins of bones of the vertebral column, the internal and external vertebral plexuses form Batson's plexus (Domisse, 1975). These veins are predominantly in the antero-lateral part of the epidural space, and ultimately drain into the azygous system of veins. As the whole system is valveless, increased intrathoracic or intra-abdominal pressure (e.g. ascites, pregnancy) can lead to major congestion and vessel enlargement within the spinal canal. The epidural venous plexus is surrounded by sparse quantity of fat.

The anterior epidural space is entirely occupied by a rich venous plexus (valveless system of veins). The plexus communicates with the intracranial sigmoid, basilar venous sinuses, basivertebral vein, occipital vein, and the azygous system. The plexus is linked to the abdominal and thoracic veins by the intervertebral foramina and through this connection transmit intraabdominal and intrathoracic pressure to the epidural space. The rich venous plexus is also connected to the iliac veins through the sacral venous plexus. Obstruction of the inferior vena cava, advanced pregnancy or intraabdominal tumors can cause distension of the venous plexus leading to an increased risk of being traumatized during needle and/or catheter placement in the epidural space.

3.6.4 Epidural arteries

The epidural arteries located in the lumbar region of the vertebral column are branches of the ilio-lumbar arteries. These arteries are found in the lateral region of the space and therefore not threatened by an advancing epidural needle.

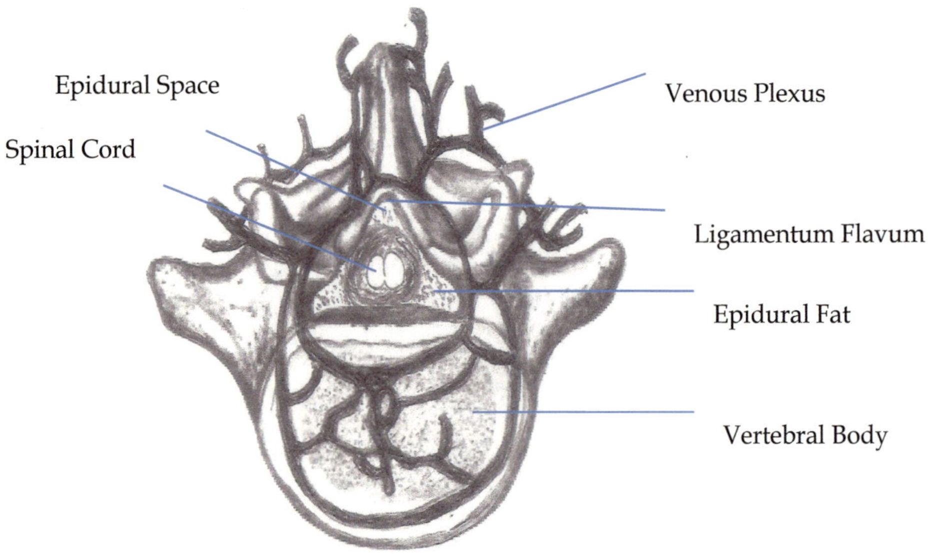

Transverse Section of Lumbar Region at L1

4. Identification of the epidural space

Identification of the epidural space is of crucial importance as it is technically demanding. The first demonstration of this space was about 78 years ago (Dogliotti, 1933). The accuracy in the location of the space however, determines the functionality of the epidural analgesia. The epidural needle, if inserted in the midline, pierces the skin and traverses the subcutaneous tissue, supraspinous ligament, interspinous ligament and through the ligamentum flavum to reach the space. The depth of the epidural space has been defined as the distance from overlying skin to the tip of the needle just penetrating into the epidural space (Lai et al., 2005). The depth can pose some difficulties during the location of the epidural space particularly in the obese patient.

To improve the success rate, the distance from skin to the epidural space and its correlation with body mass index (BMI) have been studied (Ravi et al., 2011). This study showed that as the BMI increased, the depth of the epidural space increased significant. The study was based on a predictive equation of depth of epidural space from skin in relation to BMI based on linear regression analysis as: Depth (mm) = a + b (BMI). Where a = 17.7966 and b = 0.9777.

4.1 Methods of identification

Various methods have been used in identifying the epidural space. Most of these traditional methods of locating the epidural space depend on the negative pressure exhibited during the introduction of the epidural needle into the space. Any techniques identifying the epidural space should be simple and straightforward, effective, safe, and reliable to minimize the number of complications associated with it.

One of the most reliable methods in identifying the space depends on loss of resistance (LOR). This method of identification uses either air or a liquid such as saline or a local anesthetic to achieve it. The technique applies continuous or intermittent pressure on the piston of an epidural glass or plastic syringe towards the barrel, and the loss of resistance is where it becomes possible to inject through the syringe attached to the epidural needle, so the piston can easily move into the barrel. This technique works because the ligamentum flavum is extremely dense, and injection into it is almost impossible. The syringe may contain air or saline. The principles are the same, but the specifics of the technique are different due to the greater compressibility of air with respect to saline or lidocaine.

The identification of the epidural space with LOR to air has been found to be more difficult and caused more dural punctures than with lidocaine or air plus lidocaine techniques. Additionally, sequential use of air and lidocaine had no advantage over lidocaine alone (Evron et al., 2004). The techniques of LOR to air or saline are also associated with some complications. While LOR to air has been linked to paraplegia (Nay et al., 1993), pneumocephalus (Nafiu & Bullough, 2007), LOR to saline is frequently associated with dilution of the injected local anesthetic (Okutomi & Hoka, 1998).

The epidural space has also been identified using a modified drip method (Michel & Lawes, 1991). In this study, a saline infusion was prepared, leaving the distal 40 cm of infusion tubing full of air, and then attached to the hub of a Tuohy needle. Accurate identification of the epidural space was accomplished in less than one minute in 95% of cases. This technique showed some advantages over the hanging drop and the manual loss of resistance techniques.

A technique described as "Membrane in Syringe" has been described (Lin et al., 2002). This is a modification of the loss of resistance technique for identifying the epidural space during epidural anesthesia. A plastic membrane is placed halfway inside a syringe dividing the syringe into two compartments. The saline compartment encompasses the nozzle of the syringe (the distal compartment). The plunger is installed in the opposite half of the hallow cylinder. Air is trapped in the space between the membrane and the rubber plunger (air compartment). Lin et al described this technique as having a two-fold advantage. Firstly when the syringe is filled with both normal saline and air, it can prevent injection of the air into the epidural space during identification while at the same time it does not molest the feel of compressibility. Secondly, with the membrane separating the normal saline and air, correct placement of the needle tip can also be ascertained with loss of resistance while, as will be seen, the plastic membrane will wrinkle when saline is released into the epidural space.

A clinical experience with Macintosh epidural balloon in identifying the epidural space has also been described (Fyneface-Ogan & Mato, 2008). The study compared the identification characteristics between the use of LOR to air and the epidural balloon. It showed that epidural space was identified more often at the first attempt, and more swiftly, with the epidural balloon than the LOR to air (having a greater propensity for accidental dural puncture). Though cost implication of the use of epidural balloon is more than the LOR to air, it obviously offered better advantage over the traditional use of air.

The use of Epidrum®, an optimal pressure, loss of resistance device has been described for the identification of the epidural space (Samada et al., 2011). This device is designed to operate at a high enough pressure to discharge into the epidural space but a low enough pressure to minimise premature leaking into the patients' tissues. The optimal pressure is generated by the extremely thin diaphragm on top of the device that acts as the meniscus of a manometer, so allowing the operator to interpret the diaphragm's signal to identify the position of the tip of the needle. Epidrum has been known to offer the following benefits:

- Relatively simple (offering shorter training periods). The trainer can monitor the signal when the trainee is performing the procedure
- It is safe, effective and reliable
- It allows the use of a smaller needle to: reduce post dural puncture headache and reduce epidural haematoma formation
- It offers a visual endpoint
- Optimised, low, constant pressure - minimizes false positive error
- Easily observed cerebral spinal fluid (CSF) in the event of a dural tap

Samada et al showed that Tuohy needle control was significantly easier in the Epidrum group than in the control group and concluded that Epidrum is very useful in performing epidural space identification quickly while obtaining good Tuohy needle control.

The Episure syringe® has been described as a useful tool in the identification of the epidural space (Riley & Carvalho, 2007). This is a unique spring-loaded loss-of-resistance (LOR) syringe with a coaxial compression spring within a Portex Pulsator® LOR syringe. This syringe supplies a constant pressure while the operator is advancing the Tuohy needle.

One application for this syringe may be to facilitate teaching of the epidural technique to clinicians. Both the student and the teacher will get an objective, visual signal when the needle tip enters the epidural space. The spring-loaded syringe may assist attending physicians in more closely supervising residents doing an essentially "blind," subjective procedure. While it has been extensively recommended as a useful tool in epidural space identification (Riley & Carvalho, 2007), another group of workers (Habib et al., 2008) showed that the episure syringe did not appear to have major disadvantages over the standard glass syringe amongst parturients.

One study (Rodiera et al., 1995) demonstrated the use of a mathematical analysis in identifying the epidural space. In this study pressure variations within an injection system during the epidural puncture were measured and pressure curves analyzed for amplitude and rate of decay after entry of the needle into the epidural space. The study showed that pressure changes were observed as the epidural needle traversed the skin, subcutaneous fat and muscle. The change in pressure observed when the needle entered the epidural space fitted a negative exponential function. In the study, Rodiera et al concluded that pressures within the injection system for epidural puncture can rise as high as 1100 cmH_2O. The location of the space is characterized by an exponential decay to an end-residual pressure below 50 cm H_2O.

Another method of objective identification of the epidural space for correct needle placement has been suggested (Ghelber et al., 2008). This study evaluated continuous pressure measurement during low speed injection with a computerized injection pump to locate the epidural space.

Neuraxial ultrasonography is a recent development in regional anesthesia practice particularly in epidural space identification (Perlas, 2010). Most clinical studies and data however, emanate from very few centres with highly skilled operators. It is a useful adjunct to physical examination, allowing for a highly precise identification of regional landmarks and a precise estimation of epidural space depth, thus facilitating epidural catheter insertion.

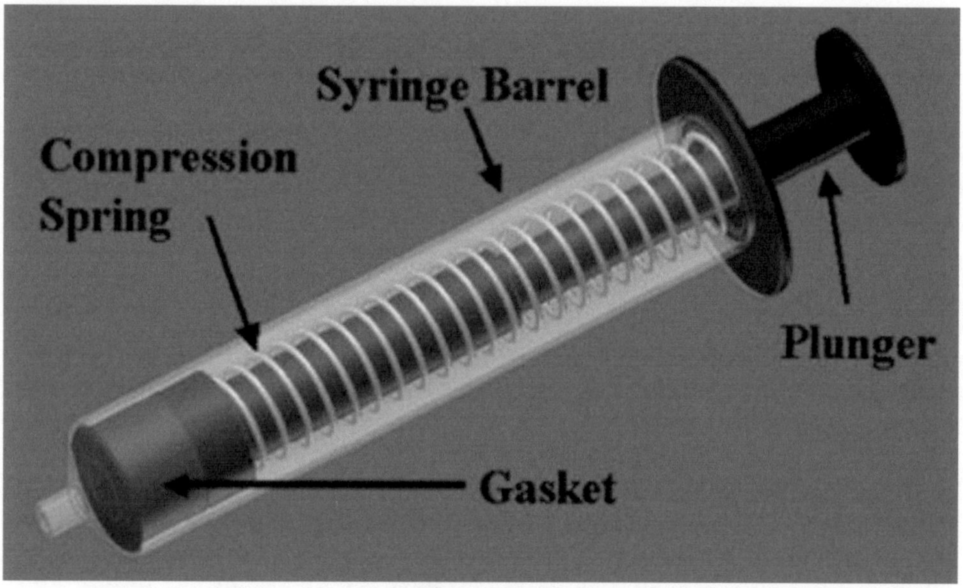

The Episure Syringe

One of such ultrasonographic studies has been shown to facilitate accurate identification of the intervertebral level and to predict skin-to-epidural depth in the lumbar epidural space with reliable precision (Rasoulian et al., 2011). A pre-puncture ultrasound for localization of the thoracic epidural space measuring the skin-to-epidural depth has been shown to correlate with the actual depth observed during epidural catheterization (Rasoulian et al., 2011). This study showed that the limits of agreement are wide, which restricts the predictive value of ultrasound-based measurements.

The use of imaging techniques has also involved the application of Magnetic Resonance Imaging (MRI) in the epidural space identification. One study has shown that the use of ultrasound showed good correlation with MRI, which is a standard imaging technique for the depiction of the spine (Grau et al., 2011). Generally, the epidural space is variable in size along its length. The space between the C7 and T1 is relatively consistent and prominent in size. A sagittal MRI with T1 sequencing is frequently known by bright signal displayed by the epidural fat in the space.

5. Clinical importance of the epidural space

The epidural space has been subjected to many clinical manipulations for purposes of anesthesia and analgesia. Injection into this space can be by a single shot, intermittent, continuous or under the control of the patient (Patient controlled epidural analgesia (PCEA)). Intermittent or continuous injections into the space are carried out through an epidural catheter. The epidural space is catheterized in a wide range of clinical reasons.

5.1 Epidural space steroid injection

Epidural injection of corticosteroids is one of the most commonly used interventions in managing radicular pain caused by nerve irritation (Mulligan & Rowlingson, 2001). Steroids placed in the epidural space have a very potent anti-inflammatory action that can decrease pain and allow patients to improve function. Although steroids do not change the underlying condition, they can break the cycle of pain and inflammation and, allow the body to compensate for the condition.

5.2 Labor and postoperative pain management

The administration of local anesthetics with or without opioids into the epidural space provides and maintains pain relief during labor, abdominal surgery, pelvis or lower limb. It is also used for pain management in conditions associated with chronic pain (including back pain, and palliation for intractable pain of neoplastic origin). It has also been found useful in the extension of regional anesthesia/analgesia during prolonged intraoperative period.

6. Conclusion

A good knowledge of the anatomy of the epidural space is imperative in the exploration of this space. The identification of this space demands some skill due to its complexity. Inadequate knowledge of the anatomy of the space and lack of skill to identify it can expose the patient to avoidable hazards such as accidental dural puncture. The dural puncture in turn leads to intractable headache following cerebrospinal fluid leakage and traction on the meninges.

The space has been manipulated in several ways for the purposes of anesthesia, analgesia and drug treatment such as steroid injection. The space, when catheterized, has been used to prolong pain relief and regional anesthesia intraoperatively. Its importance in postoperative pain management cannot be under-emphasized.

7. Conflict of interest

None.

8. Acknowledgement

I thank Mrs. Gloria Sotonye-Ogan for the excellent secretarial work in preparing this manuscript.

9. References

Blomberg RG & Olsson SS. (1989). The lumbar epidural space in patients examined with epiduroscopy. *Anesthesia & Analgesia*, Vol. 68, pp. (157-160)

Brockstein B, Johns L & Gewertz BL. (1994). Blood supply to the spinal cord: anatomic and physiologic correlations. *Ann Vasc Surg*, Vol. 8, pp. (394 -399)

Bromage, PR. (1978). Epidural analgesia. Philadelphia: WB Saunders, pp. 191–196.

Corning, JL. (1885). Spinal anesthesia and local medication of the cord. *N Y Med J*, Vol. 42, p. (483)

Danelli G, Ghisi D, Bellinghieri F, Borghi B, Fanelli G & Chelly JE. (2011). The nerve stimulation technique versus the loss of resistance technique for the posterior approach to lumbar plexus block: a randomized, prospective, observer-blinded, pilot study. *Minerva Anestesiologica,* Vol. 77, pp. (959-963)

Dogliotti AM. (1933). Research and clinical observations on spinal anaesthesia: with special reference to the peridural technique. *Anesthesia & Analgesia,* Vol. 12, pp. (59-65)

Domisse GF. (1975). The arteries and veins of the human spinal cord from birth. Edinburgh: Churchill Livingstone. pp. (81-96)

Evron S, Sessler D, Sadan O, Boaz M, Glezerman M & Ezri T. (2004). Identification of the Epidural Space: Loss of Resistance with Air, Lidocaine, or the Combination of Air and Lidocaine. *Anesthesia & Analgesia,* Vol. 99, pp. (245-250)

Fyneface-Ogan S & Mato CN. (2008). A clinical experience with epidural balloon in the localization of the epidural space in laboring parturients. *Nig Q J Hosp Med,* Vol. 18, pp. (166-169)

Ghelber O, Gebhard RE, Vora S, Hagberg CA & Szmuk P. (2008). Identification of the epidural space using pressure measurement with the compuflo injection pump - a pilot study. *Reg Anesth Pain Med,* Vol. 33, pp. (346-352)

Gil NS, Lee JH, Yoon SZ, Jeon Y, Lim YJ & Bahk JH. (2008). Comparison of thoracic epidural pressure in the sitting and lateral decubitus positions. *Anesthesiology,* Vol. 109, pp. (67-71).

Grau T, Leipold RW, Delorme S, Martin E & Motsch J. (2002). Ultrasound imaging of the thoracic epidural space. *Reg Anesth Pain Med,* Vol. 27, pp. (200-206)

Habib AS, George RB, Allen TK & Olufolabi AJ. (2008). Pilot Study to Compare the Episure® Autodetect® Syringe with the Glass Syringe for Identification of the Epidural Space in Parturients. *Anesthesia & Analgesia,* Vol. 106, pp. (541-543)

Hamid M, Fallet-Bianco C, Delmas V & Plaisant O. (2002).The human lumbar anterior epidural space: morphological comparison in adult and fetal specimens. *Surg Radiol Anat* Vol. 24, pp. (194-200)

Hogan, QH. (1991). Lumbar epidural anatomy: a new look by cryomicrotome section. *Anesthesiology,* Vol. 75, pp. (767-775)

Hogan QH. (1998). Epidural anatomy: new observations. *Can J Anaesth,* Vol. 45, pp. (40-48)

Husemeyer RP & White DC. (1980). Topography of the lumbar epidural space. A study in cadavers using injected polyester resin. *Anaesthesia,* Vol 35, pp. (7-11)

Lai HC, Liu TJ, Peng SK, Lee KC, Luk HN & Lee SC. (2005). Depth of the thoracic epidural space in paramedian approach. *J Clin Anaesth,* Vol. 17, pp. (339-343)

Lin BC, Chen KB, Chang CS, Wu KC, Liu YC, Chen CC & Wu RS. (2002). A 'membrane in syringe' technique that allows identification of the epidural space with saline while avoids injection of air into the epidural space. *Acta Anaesthesiol Sin,* Vol. 40, pp. (55-60)

Mackintosh, RR.; & Lee, JA. (1973). Lumbar puncture and spinal analgesia, Churchill Livingstone. 3rd ed. ISBN 0-443-00997-X

Mehl AL. (1986). Interpretation of traumatic lumbar puncture. *Clin Pediatr* Vol. 25, pp. (523-526)

Michel MZ & Lawes EG. (1991). Identification of epidural space by drip method. *Reg Anesth,* Vol. 16, pp. (236-239)

Mulligan KA & Rowlingson JC. (2001). Epidural steroids. *Curr Pain Headache Rep,* Vol. 5, pp. (495-502)

Nafiu OO & Bullough AS. (2007). Pneumocephalus and Headache After Epidural Analgesia: Should We Really Still Be Using Air? Anesthesia & Analgesia, Vol. 105, pp. (1172-1173)

Nay PG, Milaszkiewicz R & Jothilingam S. (1993). Extradural air as a cause of paraplegia following lumbar analgesia. *Anaesthesia*, Vol. 48, pp. (402- 404)

Nickallis RWD & Kokri MS. (1986). The width of posterior epidural space in obstetric patients. *Anaesthesia*, Vol. 41 pp. (432-433)

Okutomi T & Hoka S. (1998). Epidural saline solution prior to local anaesthetic produces differential nerve block. *Can J Anaesth* Vol. 45, pp. (1091-1093)

Parkin IG & Harrison GR. (1985). The topographical anatomy of the lumbar epidural space. *Journal of Anatomy*, Vol. 141, pp. (211-217)

Perlas A. (2010). Evidence for the use of ultrasound in neuraxial blocks. *Reg Anesth Pain Med*, Vol. 35, pp. (S43-46)

Rasoulian A, Lohser J, Najafi M, Rafii-Tari H, Tran D, Kamani AA, Lessoway VA, Abolmaesumi P & Rohling RN. (2011). Utility of prepuncture ultrasound for localization of the thoracic epidural space. *Can J Anaesth*, Vol. 58, pp. (815-823)

Ravi KK, Kaul TK, Kathuria S, Gupta S & Khurana S. (2011). Distance from skin to epidural space: Correlation with body mass index (BMI). *J Anaesthesiol Clin Pharm*, Vol. 27, pp. (39-42)

Reina MA, Franco CD, Lopez A, De Andres JA & van Zundert A. (2009). Clinical implications of epidural fat in the spinal canal. A scanning electron microscopic study. *Acta Anesthesiol Belg*, Vol. 60, pp. (7-17)

Reina MA, Pulido P, Castedo J, Villanueva MC, López A & Sola RG. (2006). Characteristics and distribution of normal human epidural fat. *Rev Esp Anestesiol Reanim*, Vol. 53, pp. (363-372)

Riley ET & Carvalho B. (2007). The Episure™ Syringe: A Novel Loss of Resistance Syringe for Locating the Epidural Space. *Anesthesia & Analgesia*, Vol. 105, pp. (1164-1166)

Rodiera J, Calabuig R, Aliaga L, Espinosa W, Hobeich F, Oferil F & Gual A. (1995). Mathematical analysis of epidural space location. *International Journal of Clinical Monitoring and Computing, Vol. 12, pp. (213-217)*

Sawada A, Kii N, Yoshikawa Y & Yamakage M. (2011). Epidrum(®): a new device to identify the epidural space with an epidural Tuohy needle. *J Anesth* Nov 13.

Usubiaga, JE.; Moya, F & Usubiaga, LE. (1967). A note on the recording of epidural negative pressure. *Canadian Anaesthesia Society Journal*, Vol. 14, pp. (119-122)

Williams PL, Warwick R, Dyson M & Bannister LH. (1989). Gray's anatomy. 37th Ed. Edinburgh: Churchill Livingstone. pp. (1123–1143)

Yan L, Li J, Zhao W, Cui Z, Wang H & Xin L. (2010). The study of epidurography and multispiral CT scanning examinations in the diagnosis of lumbar nerve root canal stenosis. *Orthopedics*, Vol. 33, pp. (732). doi: 10.3928/01477447-20100826-05.

Zarzur, E. (1984). Genesis of the 'true' negative pressure in the lumbar epidural space: a new hypothesis. *Anaesthesia*, Vol. 39, pp. (1101-1104)

2

Local Anaesthetic Epidural Solution for Labour: About Concentrations and Additives

Christian Dualé and Martine Bonnin
CHU Clermont-Ferrand,
Centre de Pharmacologie Clinique (Inserm CIC 501),
Anesthésie-Réanimation-Estaing,
France

1. Introduction

Epidural analgesia can be considered nowadays as the standard technique to relieve pain during labour. Wide information is now available about the different parameters the clinician has to choose to conduct it, namely drugs, concentrations, regimens and additives. The recently published guidelines from the *American Society of Anesthesiologists Task Force on Obstetric Anesthesia* illustrate the strong improvement of knowledge in this field (ASA Task Force on Obstetric Anesthesia, 2007). Nevertheless, the actual research still focuses on the pathways to increase the efficacy/risk ratio of epidural analgesia.

A first option is to develop local anaesthetics with a hypothetical lower toxicity, thanks to the pharmaceutical companies for this effort. As an example, two amide local anaesthetics produced in the pure levorotatory form - ropivacaine and levobupivacaine - are now available for epidural analgesia in labour, to face the hypothetical risk of toxicity of bupivacaine. The use of ropivacaine has increased in the field of obstetrics in some industrialised countries (Beilin et al., 2007; Sah et al., 2007; Page et al., 2008; Beilin & Halpern, 2010). Levobupivacaine, the pure S(-)-enantiomer of bupivacaine, recently emerged as a safer alternative for regional anesthesia than its racemic parent (Bardsley et al., 1998; Mather & Chang, 2001; Burlacu & Buggy, 2008). In addition to a lower toxicity *per se*, levobupivacaine has been claimed by some authors to be more potent than bupivacaine (Camorcia & Capogna, 2003; Sah et al., 2007) or ropivacaine (Benhamou et al., 2003), (Burlacu & Buggy, 2008), and even to induce less impairment of motricity (Lacassie & Columb, 2003; Beilin et al., 2007; Lacassie et al., 2007; Sah et al., 2007).

A second option is to lower the concentration of the local anaesthetic solution. This option would somewhat mitigate the problem of bupivacaine toxicity, and may also explain why a superior safety of the two recent molecules is not yet clinically evidenced. The practice of epidural analgesia for labour in our institution - a university hospital of central France in which about 3.500 women deliver yearly - may illustrate this issue. Indeed, the protocols in for induction and maintenance of analgesia the early 80's used top-up injections of bupivacaine 0.25%, or even more in some cases. Analgesia seemed excellent for most of the parturients, but with this practice raised also questions about side effects, namely impairment of motricity and proprioception. Practitioners were therefore questioned by a publication of Chestnut et al. (Chestnut et al., 1988), reporting the interest of an infusion of bupivacaine, i.e. four times less concentrated than in their practice. This highlighted the virtues of the differential nerve block, with a possibility to block selectively the nociceptive pathways (i.e. unmyelinated or few myelinated fibres) without affecting the other components of nerve transmission (Powell et al., 1988; Reid, 1998). Practitioners were therefore encouraged to use a new range of concentrations, from the lowest (i.e. 0.0625 to 0.08%), to higher - but reasonable - concentrations (around 0.125%). The aim was to strike a difficult balance between the lowest motor block possible (to facilitate labour and vaginal delivery, and even allow ambulation) and an optimal analgesia (Polley et al., 2003; Benhamou et al., 2003; ASA Task Force on Obstetric Anesthesia, 2007; Buyse et al., 2007). Fortunately, the risk of a failure of analgesia with the lowest concentrations could be reduced by the systematic adjunction of epidural opiates (Bernard et al., 2001; Benhamou et al., 2002; Halpern et al., 2003; Lim et al., 2004; ASA Task Force on Obstetric Anesthesia, 2007; Mcleod et al., 2007). Interestingly, it seems that such potentiation by epidural opiates is due to a segmental action, as opiates are able to reduce the minimal local anaesthetic concentration (MLAC) (Polley et al., 1998; Robinson et al., 2001; Ginosar et al., 2003; Buyse et al., 2007).

Since then, it appears that many physicians have reduced the current concentrations in their daily practice. In our hospital for example, a 0.125%-concentration is now the maximal standard for bupivacaine, while ropivacaine and levobupivacaine are preferred by some practitioners. However, it seems that the concentration issue is still incompletely resolved and needs further investigation. This was highlighted in 2007 with two interesting statements of the ASA Task Force (ASA Task Force on Obstetric Anesthesia, 2007):

1. There are no differences in the analgesic efficacy of low concentrated solutions with opiates, compared with higher concentrations without opiates (the cut-off value for concentration being bupivacaine 0.125% or equivalent). However, it is not known if this level of analgesic efficacy can be considered as optimal, or if it could be improved. Would such equivalence still exist if low concentrated solutions with opiates were compared to higher concentrations with opiates? Is the use of higher concentrations also completely safe, in terms of drug income?
2. The technique to select "should reflect patient needs and preferences, practitioner preferences or skills, and available resources" (ASA Task Force on Obstetric Anesthesia, 2007). Although anyone would agree with this wise recommendation, the issue of preference(s) probably needs clarification. Are there standard - and evidenced-based - criteria on which can be determined either the patient's, or the practitioner's preference between two or more techniques?

A good illustration of the issue is the marketing of levobupivacaine in France, which, since July 2005, is available in pre-filled bags (100 or 200 mL) with two different concentrations (0.625 and 1.25 $mg.mL^{-1}$). Both presentations have the same indication, i.e. analgesia in postoperative context and in labour (AFSSAPS, 2011a; AFSSAPS, 2011b). Then, the choice between the two concentrations mostly depends on the practitioner, and this choice appears to depend mostly of his/her personal beliefs, rather than of scientific evidence. Furthermore, the parturient may not be very often implicated in such decision, especially if the respective expected effects of both techniques cannot be clearly described to her.

2. Comparing two concentrations, both with opiates

Our aim was to give an answer to the question of equivalence between a low concentrated solution with opiates, and higher concentrations, also with opiates. We also wanted to keep quite pragmatic conditions, to help the practitioners in their practice. For this, we chose the two presentations of levobupivacaine in pre-filled bags (see above), as our institution was quite familiar with these. We felt the pre-filled bags were very convenient for our protocols of epidural analgesia, as the solution could be used for induction and patient-controlled maintenance, the syringe being refilled without hazardous manipulation.

We planned a randomised, controlled and double-blinded trial (see ClinicalTrials.gov NCT00929682, and (Tixier et al., 2010)).

The aim of the trial was to compare the two available presentations of levobupivacaine, in conditions the closest possible to our daily practice. In one arm, the solution for epidural analgesia was levobupivacaine 0.0625% (called LC for low concentration), in the other, it was levobupivacaine 0.125% (called HC for high concentration). In each 100-mL prefilled bag of solution, 10 mL (50 μg) of sufentanil were added. Opiates were also used in the HC group to assess the effect of concentration, without interaction. The final concentrations of levobupicaine were 0.568 or 1.136 $mg.mL^{-1}$, with sufentanil 0.45 $\mu g.mL^{-1}$.

The prepared solutions were used both for the induction and the maintenance of analgesia. Induction of analgesia with an initial volume of 20 mL of anaesthetic solution, followed by a standardised algorithm of top-up manual injections to achieve analgesia, then by a patient-controlled regimen with 5-mL self-administered boli in addition to a continuous infusion of 5 $mL.hr^{-1}$. Our choice for this regimen was a compromise between efficacy and risks (Ferrante et al., 1994; Lim et al., 2008; Halpern & Carvalho, 2009). Manual injections were always performed by an anaesthetist, with a separate syringe directly filled from the solution bag, after disinfection of the sites. To refill the syringe of the patient-controlled epidural analgesia (PCEA) device, the solution was drawn from the bag through a parallel line secured by a three-way tap.

The study included women in spontaneous uncomplicated labour, with cervical dilatation ≤ 7 cm. We included only primiparous women, because pain during labour is commonly more resistant to relief in this sub-population, so we could sort out a greater effect size, and also to increase homogeneity beneath the sample. We excluded induced labour with the same aim of homogeneity, even if this condition is supposed to increase pain during contractions. Indeed, medical induction of labour was not a frequent practice in our centre, and it was simpler to exclude these patients, rather than to plan a stratified randomisation. We also excluded breech presentation, overweight, multiple pregnancy, preeclampsia, or any fetal abnormality.

The principal objective of the study was to assess the quality of the analgesia provided by the two different concentrations of levobupivacaine. As the protocol chosen associated a PCEA and many levels of rescue administration, we were not expecting to observe a difference in the quality of analgesia, but we hypothesised that greater amounts of solution would be administered in the LC group. However, we kept the quality of analgesia as a secondary endpoint. The sample size was estimated from data we had from a previous trial undertaken in our unit in 59 parturients having had a patient-controlled epidural analgesia for labour with 0.125% bupivacaine plus sufentanil 0.25 μg.mL^{-1} (Vernis et al., 2004). Fifty-seven patients per group were necessary to identify a 25% difference in the primary endpoint, i.e. the hourly consumption of the analgesic solution in mL.hr^{-1}. This number was reached, with 65 patients in the LC group and 60 in the HC group.

Contrary to our expectations, and this probably due to the PCEA regimen, the quality of analgesia was superior in the HC group. The following table illustrates the size of this effect of superiority, i.e. the percentage of reduction of the mean value for the outcome, from LC to HC. The effect size is here calculated out of the mean values in each group. The p value was < 0.05 for all the comparisons of outcomes, between the two groups.

Outcome	Effect size
Pain score 30 minutes after induction	-30%
Nb. of observations with pain score > 3/10, 30 minutes after induction	-65%
Pain amount (area under curve) during the first 3 hours after induction	-23%
Percentage (per patient) of observations with pain score > 3/10	-46%
Pain score at expulsion	-48%
Pain score at suture of episiotomy or tear	-61%

We chose this cut-off level of 3/10 to define the cases of relevant pain, as (i) this value is considered as the superior limit of the definition for mild pain (Breivik et al., 2008), and (ii) satisfaction is usually good to excellent when pain scores stay below this level (Halpern et al., 2003).

Probably because of the regimen of administration chosen, this difference in analgesic efficacy was associated to more self- and medically administered epidural injections in the LC group. This analysis considered only the patients who had vaginal delivery (n = 58 and 49 in the LC and HC group, respectively). The following table illustrates the size of this effect, as previously described.

Outcome	Effect size
Nb. of patient-administered boluses	-37%
Required volume of epidural infusion (in ml.hr^{-1})	-20%

We unfortunately did not assess the patient's satisfaction in this study, believing it was not an outcome easy to interpret. It is therefore difficult to know if the observed difference in the quality of analgesia was relevant, as – for example – the percentage (per patient) of observations with pain score > 3/10 was quite low (20%) even in the LC group. This issue led us to reconsider the systematic assessment of the patient's satisfaction for further trials, even if this outcome is rarely studied in the trials about analgesia for labour.

Considering safety, we did not find any difference between the two groups for all the outcomes that could be considered as expected side effects of epidural analgesia for labour, namely motor effects, effects on labour and foetal outcomes. However, this must always been considered with caution, as such small-sample studies are always underpowered to sort out such differences. To improve the power to detect an impairment of normal delivery, we created a composite binary outcome defined by the occurrence of one of these two outcomes: a caesarean section or a labour lasting more than 390 min, this cut-off value being the third quartile of the whole duration of labour in the subgroup of parturients with vaginal delivery. The risk for this composite outcome was the same in the two groups (37 and 38% in the LC and HC group, respectively).

We noted however that in the HC group, the administered dose of levobupivacaine overstepped the French recommendations (12.5 $mg.hr^{-1}$) in more than 1/3 of the cases (AFSSAPS, 2011a; AFSSAPS, 2011b), while this never occurred in the LC group. This had no clinical consequences, probably because these French limits are much lower than the possibly toxic dose in humans (Burlacu & Buggy, 2008; Purdue Pharma, 2011).

To summarise, we noted particular points in these results:

1. the low-concentrated solution - even with opiates - provided analgesia of lower quality, although we did not assess the impact on the patients' satisfaction;
2. the low-concentrated solution with added opiates provided an excellent analgesia, but the doses administered were often quite high, although we were not potent enough to assess the real clinical effects of such overdosage.

At this step of our reflexion, we felt that two options appeared to increase the efficacy/risk ratio of epidural analgesia for labour:

1. to develop an intermediate concentration, to which opiates should be added;
2. to make ourselves this solution with an intermediate concentration, with the obvious inconveniences of a hazardous manual intervention and a higher cost;
3. to potentiate the analgesia induced by the low-concentrated solution (plus opiates) by another epidural co-analgesic.

3. Improving analgesic efficacy of low concentrated solutions

We orientated our investigation on the third choice, as we felt the opportunity to test clonidine as an additive. Clonidine was a well-known drug in our practice, with a quite old history of perispinal administration, as the first report was in 1987 in France (Racle et al., 1987). This choice was supported by the following arguments:

1. clonidine inhibits nociceptive transmission in spinal cord via α_2 receptors, and may have in addition local anaesthetic effects (Singelyn et al., 1996; Kroin et al., 2004);
2. it was - at least in France - often used epidurally for labour as single injection, either at the induction of epidural analgesia or as a rescue treatment (Chassard et al., 1996; Landau et al., 2002);
3. the systematic addition of clonidine in the solution used for epidural infusion was known to improve post-operative analgesia in diverse models (Tremlett et al., 1999; Paech et al., 2000; Kayacan et al., 2004; Parker et al., 2007);
4. already two French studies used levobupivacaine 0.0625% given on PCEA with low-concentrated clonidine, with promising results (Fontaine et al., 2008; Wallet et al., 2010);
5. we recently evidenced the stability over 24 hours of a solution in which levobupivacaine, sufentanil and clonidine were mixed together (Sautou et al., 2011).

We then planned a second randomised, controlled and double-blinded trial (see ClinicalTrials.gov NCT00983125, and (Bazin et al., 2011)).

To propose a protocol simple to apply, we thought that adding 150 µg of clonidine to the LC solution previously studied, would provide a quality of analgesia close to which was given by the HC solution, without the inconvenience of this latter. The two treatments to be compared were then:

- in one arm, levobupivacaine 0.0625% plus sufentanil (0.45 $\mu g.ml^{-1}$) plus 150 µg of clonidine,
- in the other arm, the same solution with no clonidine.

The final concentration of clonidine was 1.35 $\mu g.ml^{-1}$. The control group was then very similar to the LC group in the previous study (Tixier et al., 2010).

The choice of this dose of clonidine was motivated by the two following arguments:

1. a safety issue, as this dose was in the range for which a co-analgesic effect had been found with no increase of side effects (Tremlett et al., 1999; Kayacan et al., 2004; Huang et al., 2007; Fontaine et al., 2008);
2. practical reasons, as it seemed easy to the practitioner to add the full dose of the available presentation of clonidine (150 µg) to the prefilled bag of levobupivacaine at the start of epidural analgesia.

The volumes used and the maintenance regimens (PCEA) were similar to those used in the previous study (Tixier et al., 2010). The inclusion and non-inclusion criteria were also the same, except the required cervical dilatation set to ≤ 5 cm. The primary outcome was the total number of additional boluses, i.e. either self-administered or manually administered by the anaesthetist as a rescue.

The sample size estimation was based on the values for the primary outcome that were noted in the previous study (Tixier et al., 2010). As clonidine was not labelled for epidural administration during labour in France, we planned interim analyses, to be able to discontinue the trial in case of safety problems. The initial objective (62 patients per group) was reached (125 patients included), but 10 protocol violations occurred; the effects on the primary outcome were anyway analysed in intent-to-treat.

The superiority of the solution with added clonidine compared to the control was evidenced, for all the outcomes related to the quality of analgesia. Here, we analysed the effects on pain by a linear mixed model, which showed a significant difference ($p < 0.0001$ for the model), with an effect of time and of interaction treatment*time. Furthermore, even satisfaction was greater in the clonidine group ($p = 0.0006$), which is not often noted in such trials. The superiority was also noted for most of the outcomes related to consumption of the epidural solution.

The following table illustrates the size of this effect of superiority, i.e. the percentage of reduction of the mean value for the outcome, from placebo group to clonidine group. The effect size is here calculated out of the mean values in each group. The p value was < 0.05 for all the comparison of outcomes, between the two groups.

Considering the hourly administered dose of levobupivacaine, the level recommended by the French label for the drug (12.5 $mg.hr^{-1}$) was overstepped in only one case, in the placebo group (AFSSAPS, 2011a; AFSSAPS, 2011b).

Outcome	**Effect size**
Pain score 30 minutes after induction	-37%
Nb. of observations with pain score > 3/10, 30 minutes after induction	-59%
Pain amount (area under curve) during the first 3 hours after induction	-36%
Percentage (per patient) of observations with pain score > 3/10	-70%
Pain score at expulsion	-67%
Pain score at suture of episiotomy or tear	-52%
Nb. of patient-administered boluses	-35%
Required volume of epidural infusion (in $ml.hr^{-1}$)	-15%

Epidural clonidine is likely to induce dose-dependent side effects:

- maternal sedation (O'Meara & Gin, 1993; Paech et al., 2000; Aveline et al., 2002; Gurses et al., 2003; Roelants et al., 2005);
- maternal hypotension (Chassard et al., 1996; Landau et al., 2002; Aveline et al., 2002; Gurses et al., 2003; Roelants et al., 2005; Parker et al., 2007; Wallet et al., 2010);
- maternal bradycardia (O'Meara & Gin, 1993; Gurses et al., 2003; Huang et al., 2007);
- abnormalities in foetal heart rhythm (Chassard et al., 1996; Tremlett et al., 1999).

In addition, its intrinsic properties to act as a blocker of nerve transmission (Kroin et al., 2004) could in theory have deleterious effects on labour, as it would be expected with a high-concentrated local anaesthetic agent.

Probably due to the dose chosen, we did not observe serious adverse event in the clonidine group; nevertheless, there was a clear effect of clonidine on maternal blood pressure, uncorrelated to the quality of analgesia. We noted also a highest rate of instrumental delivery in the clonidine group (35 vs. 18%, $p = 0.042$). As such pilot studies are underpowered for the infrequently positive outcomes, no conclusion about safety can be given. However, for the composite outcome we created to represent the impairment of normal delivery (see above), the risk was not superior in the clonidine group (37% vs. 53%, n.s.).

At this stage, it seemed interesting to compare side by side the results of our two studies (four groups), according to the fact that two groups (one from each study) had basically the same analgesic protocol (i.e. levobupivacaine 0.0625% + 50 µg of sufentanil), and the two other groups provided a superior analgesia compared to this protocol. The following table next page helps for this comparison, which remains intentionally descriptive (the values shown are the median).

Study	(Tixier et al., 2010)	(Bazin et al., 2011)	(Tixier et al., 2010)	(Bazin et al., 2011)
Concentration of levobupivacaine [a]	0.0625%	0.0625%	0.125%	0.0625%
Added sufentanil [b]	50 µg	50 µg	50 µg	50 µg
Added clonidine [b]	None	None	None	150 µg
Pain after induction [c,d]	3	3	2	2
Relevant pain after induction [d,e]	35%	29%	14%	12%
Pain amount [f]	8.8	8.3	6.5	4.3
Time spent with relevant pain [e,g]	20%	33%	11%	10%
Pain at expulsion [c,h]	3	5	1	0
Pain at suture of episiotomy or tear [c,h]	2	3	0	0
Number of patient-administered boluses	8.5	9	6	6
Number of rescue injections [i]	0.2	0.1	0.3	0.3
Required volume of epidural infusion [j]	13	13	10	10

Notes: a Initial concentration, i.e. solution in the prefilled bag.
b Initial full dose, added to the initial solution in the prefilled bag.
c Pain score measured on visual analogue scale (VAS), out of 10.
d Measured 30 minutes after the induction of the epidural analgesia.
e An observation of relevant pain is an observation of a pain score superior to 3/10 on the visual analogue scale. Here is expressed a rate of positive observations (one per patient) out of the whole group.
f This is the area under curve for the pain scores measured on VAS, calculated for the first 3 hours after induction according to the trapezoidal rule (Vernis et al., 2004). Patients with missing data (because of early delivery) are excluded.
g Here is calculated, for each patient, the rate of observations with relevant pain, out of the total number of observations (one per hour throughout labour).
h I.e. medically administered as a rescue, during maintenance of analgesia. Here are expressed the mean values, all the median values being equal to 0.
i Expressed in $ml.hr^{-1}$.

A systematic addition of clonidine to a low-concentrated solution of local anaesthetic could be therefore a very interesting option, as this may provide the same quality of analgesia than with high-concentrated, but with much lower amounts of anaesthetic given. However, the safety of clonidine is not fully evidenced yet.

4. New trials to improve our daily practice?

4.1 The jungle of variability

Our results provided interesting information for future research. It would be interesting, for example, to compare a low-concentrated local anaesthetic plus clonidine, with a high-concentrated solution (both having an opiate in addition).

The encouraging results obtained from these pilot studies may not be sufficient to result in a change of the current practice in obstetrical analgesia. The main reason for this is the small size of these trials, which does not allow concluding, for example, to the full safety of an epidural infusion of a local anaesthetic solution in which clonidine would be added in a systematic way. It is widely accepted that large-sized, pragmatic trials are mandatory to reach a high level of evidence and to influence the medical practice. Such trials are especially tricky to develop in the field of analgesia for labour, because of the huge variability observed at different levels.

Variability in the strategies to rule out epidural analgesia for labour. This is obvious in the published studies, as well as in the current practice of the centres. Multiple elements are to be considered in these strategies, such as:

- the level of puncture;
- the protocol of induction;
- the drug its concentration and the additional opiates (sometimes different for induction and for maintenance);
- the respective roles of the parturient (PCEA…) and the practitioner(s);
- the protocol of maintenance (top-up injections, continuous infusion…)…

Variability in the obstetrical conditions. Three particular conditions are known to increase the intensity of pain during labour, and therefore to reduce the efficacy of analgesic strategies:

- nulliparity,
- medically-induced labour,
- advanced stage of labour.

Variability in the obstetrical practice. The assessment of a new strategy in a validation controlled trial, for example a systematic addition of clonidine to the current epidural solution, would need a sensible assessment of safety outcomes. Some of them, such as motricity, maternal and foetal haemodynamics or sedation level, may be influenced by the new strategy alone. The obstetrical outcomes, such as the duration of labour, the rate of instrumental delivery and the rate of caesarean section, are likely to be also influenced by the obstetrical practice, which varies with the centre, the country, and the year (Ecker & Frigoletto, Jr., 2007; Sufang et al., 2007). Furthermore, analgesia itself may interact with some of them, as for example a better analgesia may incitate to instrumental delivery.

4.2 Modelism vs. pragmatism

Reducing variability by recruiting very homogeneous samples of patients and by standardising the anaesthetic procedures, is a very common method used in clinical research. The main advantage of such methodology is to reach statistical significance with small samples and to quantify effect sizes in very particular situations. However, the results of such studies are unlikely to influence the current practice, as the conditions of the trial may not be considered as realistic to the reader. What would be the effect of clonidine added to bupivacaine administered by top-up injections in multiparous parturients? Furthermore, some of the techniques used (new drugs, PCEA…) are not affordable in many countries.

In a pragmatic trial, we would accept variability, and this even in the choice of the molecule, as the potency of the three available local anaesthetics may be quite similar (Beilin & Halpern, 2010). In order to influence the practice worldwide, we would also accept to include patients in several countries, with all the variability in recruitment, obstetrical practice and expectations. This could be faced only by very big sample sizes, to which a stratified randomisation could be applied. The cost of such studies would be extremely high, while only academic institutions would be interested in the promotion of already labelled - or even out of patent - drugs.

4.3 What is the goal of analgesia in labour?

The gold standard for assessment of pain or analgesia is the quantification of pain on a visual analogue scale, although the numerical rating scale appears to be also a valuable tool (Hjermstad et al., 2011). This is validated in general for the post-operative context. Such outcomes may be however difficult to interpret in the context of labour, in which there may not be a strict linearity between the quality of analgesia and the feelings of the patient about the quality of care. As an example, in a large-sized study comparing epidural bupivacaine and levobupivacaine for labour in nulliparous patients, the patients were asked to quantify the quality of care at the 24th hour after delivery (Halpern et al., 2003). No difference was found between groups in the pains scores during labour. Interestingly, the patients of both groups quantified their feeling of pain relief during labour with values between 66 and 77/100 (76 for the early stage of labour), while the overall satisfaction with pain relief was higher (81/100). Furthermore, the score for the item "overall care met expectations" was even higher (89/100). This discrepancy can be easily explained by a different requirement or a greater indulgence of the patient about the quality of analgesia, to which must be added a cultural tolerance to pain during childbirth (Kloosterman, 1982).

We feel, in our practice, that the particular case of each parturient is not sufficiently considered in current practice of analgesia for labour. This is already well known for the obstetrical context (stage of labour, parity…), although more precise recommendations are still required. The issue of the patient's preferences - as abovementioned (ASA Task Force on Obstetric Anesthesia, 2007) - requires probably a better knowledge of the parturient's expectations and the predictors of her satisfaction about the treatment of labour pain.

5. Acknowledgement

We are extremely grateful to our colleagues who took part in the clinical research here mentioned, namely Marie Bazin, Franck Bolandard, Bernard Lavergne, Brigitte Storme, Sébastien Tixier and Lise Vernis, and also to Daniel Bourdeaux and Valérie Sautou (pharmacists) and Bruno Pereira (biostatistician).

6. References

AFSSAPS. CHIROCAÏNE 0,625 mg/ml, solution pour perfusion; http://afssaps-prd.afssaps.fr/php/ecodex/frames.php?specid=67913100&typedoc=R&ref=R0186626.htm . 2011a.

AFSSAPS. CHIROCAÏNE 1,25 mg/ml, solution pour perfusion; http://afssaps-prd.afssaps.fr/php/ecodex/frames.php?specid=60661814&typedoc=R&ref=R0186627.htm . 2011b.

ASA Task Force on Obstetric Anesthesia (2007). Practice guidelines for obstetric anesthesia: an updated report by the American Society of Anesthesiologists Task Force on Obstetric Anesthesia. *Anesthesiology,* Vol.106, pp.843-863.

Aveline C., El Metaoua S., Masmoudi A., Boelle P.Y., & Bonnet F. (2002). The effect of clonidine on the minimum local analgesic concentration of epidural ropivacaine during labor. *Anesthesia Analgesia,* Vol.95, pp.735-740.

Bardsley H., Gristwood R., Baker H., Watson N., & Nimmo W. (1998). A comparison of the cardiovascular effects of levobupivacaine and rac-bupivacaine following intravenous administration to healthy volunteers. *British Journal of Clinical Pharmacology,* Vol.46, pp.245-249.

Bazin M., Bonnin M., Storme B., Bolandard F., Vernis L., Lavergne B., Pereira B., Bazin J.E., & Dualé C. (2011). Addition of clonidine to a continuous patient-controlled epidural infusion of low-concentration levobupivacaine plus sufentanil in primiparous women during labour. *Anaesthesia,* Vol.66, pp.769-779.

Beilin Y., Guinn N.R., Bernstein H.H., Zahn J., Hossain S., & Bodian C.A. (2007). Local anesthetics and mode of delivery: bupivacaine versus ropivacaine versus levobupivacaine. *Anesthesia Analgesia,* Vol.105, pp.756-763.

Beilin Y., & Halpern S. (2010). Focused review: ropivacaine versus bupivacaine for epidural labor analgesia. *Anesthesia Analgesia,* Vol.111, pp.482-487.

Benhamou D., Ghosh C., & Mercier F.J. (2003). A randomized sequential allocation study to determine the minimum effective analgesic concentration of levobupivacaine and ropivacaine in patients receiving epidural analgesia for labor. *Anesthesiology,* Vol.99, pp.1383-1386.

Benhamou D., Mercier F.J., Ben Ayed M., & Auroy Y. (2002). Continuous epidural analgesia with bupivacaine 0.125% or bupivacaine 0.0625% plus sufentanil 0.25 microg.mL(-1): a study in singleton breech presentation. *International Journal of Obstetrical Anesthesia,* Vol.11, pp.13-18.

Bernard J.M., Le Roux D., Barthe A., Jourdain O., Vizquel L., & Michel C. (2001). The dose-range effects of sufentanil added to 0.125% bupivacaine on the quality of patient-controlled epidural analgesia during labor. *Anesthesia Analgesia,* Vol.92, pp.184-188.

Breivik H., Borchgrevink P.C., Allen S.M., Rosseland L.A., Romundstad L., Hals E.K., Kvarstein G., & Stubhaug A. (2008). Assessment of pain. *British Journal of Anaesthesia,* Vol.101, pp.17-24.

Burlacu C.L., & Buggy D.J. (2008). Update on local anesthetics: focus on levobupivacaine. *Therapeutics and Clinical Risk Management,* Vol.4, pp.381-392.

Buyse I., Stockman W., Columb M., Vandermeersch E., & Van de Velde M. (2007). Effect of sufentanil on minimum local analgesic concentrations of epidural bupivacaine, ropivacaine and levobupivacaine in nullipara in early labour. *International Journal of Obstetrical Anesthesia,* Vol.16, pp.22-28.

Camorcia M., & Capogna G. (2003). Epidural levobupivacaine, ropivacaine and bupivacaine in combination with sufentanil in early labour: a randomized trial. *European Journal of Anaesthesiology,* Vol.20, pp.636-639.

Chassard D., Mathon L., Dailler F., Golfier F., Tournadre J.P., & Bouletreau P. (1996). Extradural clonidine combined with sufentanil and 0.0625% bupivacaine for analgesia in labour. *British Journal of Anaesthesia,* Vol.77, pp.458-462.

Chestnut D.H., Owen C.L., Bates J.N., Ostman L.G., Choi W.W., & Geiger M.W. (1988). Continuous infusion epidural analgesia during labor: a randomized, double-blind comparison of 0.0625% bupivacaine/0.0002% fentanyl versus 0.125% bupivacaine. *Anesthesiology,* Vol.68, pp.754-759.

Ecker J.L., & Frigoletto F.D., Jr. (2007). Cesarean delivery and the risk-benefit calculus. *New England Journal of Medicine,* Vol.356, pp.885-888.

Ferrante F.M., Rosinia F.A., Gordon C., & Datta S. (1994). The role of continuous background infusions in patient-controlled epidural analgesia for labor and delivery. *Anesthesia Analgesia,* Vol.79, pp.80-84.

Fontaine M.F., Bouvet L., Long Himnam N., Page M., Dale F., Ruynat L., Chassard D., & Boselli E. (2008). [Intérêt de la clonidine en PCEA obstétricale : étude observationnelle]. *Annales Françaises d'Anesthésie et de Réanimation,* Vol.27, pp.S150.

Ginosar Y., Columb M.O., Cohen S.E., Mirikatani E., Tingle M.S., Ratner E.F., Angst M.S., & Riley E.T. (2003). The site of action of epidural fentanyl infusions in the presence of local anesthetics: a minimum local analgesic concentration infusion study in nulliparous labor. *Anesthesia Analgesia,* Vol.97, pp.1439-1445.

Gurses E., Sungurtekin H., Tomatir E., Balci C., & Gonullu M. (2003). The addition of droperidol or clonidine to epidural tramadol shortens onset time and increases duration of postoperative analgesia. *Canadian Journal of Anaesthesia,* Vol.50, pp.147-152.

Halpern S.H., Breen T.W., Campbell D.C., Muir H.A., Kronberg J., Nunn R., & Fick G.H. (2003). A multicenter, randomized, controlled trial comparing bupivacaine with ropivacaine for labor analgesia. *Anesthesiology,* Vol.98, pp.1431-1435.

Halpern S.H., & Carvalho B. (2009). Patient-controlled epidural analgesia for labor. *Anesthesia Analgesia,* Vol.108, pp.921-928.

Hjermstad M.J., Fayers P.M., Haugen D.F., Caraceni A., Hanks G.W., Loge J.H., Fainsinger R., Aass N., & Kaasa S. (2011). Studies comparing Numerical Rating Scales, Verbal Rating Scales, and Visual Analogue Scales for assessment of pain intensity in adults: a systematic literature review. *Journal of Pain and Symptom Management,* Vol.41, pp.1073-1093.

Huang Y.S., Lin L.C., Huh B.K., Sheen M.J., Yeh C.C., Wong C.S., & Wu C.T. (2007). Epidural clonidine for postoperative pain after total knee arthroplasty: a dose-response study. *Anesthesia Analgesia,* Vol.104, pp.1230-1235.

Kayacan N., Arici G., Karsli B., Bigat Z., & Akar M. (2004). Patient-controlled epidural analgesia in labour: the addition of fentanyl or clonidine to bupivacaine. *Agri,* Vol.16, pp.59-66.

Kloosterman G.J. (1982). The universal aspects of childbirth: Human birth as a socio-psychosomatic paradigm. *Journal of Psychosomatic Obstetrics and Gynaecology,* Vol.1, pp.35-41.

Kroin J.S., Buvanendran A., Beck D.R., Topic J.E., Watts D.E., & Tuman K.J. (2004). Clonidine prolongation of lidocaine analgesia after sciatic nerve block in rats is mediated via the hyperpolarization-activated cation current, not by alpha-adrenoreceptors. *Anesthesiology,* Vol.101, pp.488-494.

Lacassie H.J., & Columb M.O. (2003). The relative motor blocking potencies of bupivacaine and levobupivacaine in labor. *Anesthesia Analgesia,* Vol.97, pp.1509-1513.

Lacassie H.J., Habib A.S., Lacassie H.P., & Columb M.O. (2007). Motor blocking minimum local anesthetic concentrations of bupivacaine, levobupivacaine, and ropivacaine in labor. *Regional Anesthesia and Pain Medicine,* Vol.32, pp.323-329.

Landau R., Schiffer E., Morales M., Savoldelli G., & Kern C. (2002). The dose-sparing effect of clonidine added to ropivacaine for labor epidural analgesia. *Anesthesia Analgesia,* Vol.95, pp.728-734.

Lim Y., Ocampo C.E., Supandji M., Teoh W.H., & Sia A.T. (2008). A randomized controlled trial of three patient-controlled epidural analgesia regimens for labor. *Anesthesia Analgesia,* Vol.107, pp.1968-1972.

Lim Y., Sia A.T., & Ocampo C.E. (2004). Comparison of intrathecal levobupivacaine with and without fentanyl in combined spinal epidural for labor analgesia. *Medical Science Monitor,* Vol.10, pp.I87-I91.

Mather L.E., & Chang D.H. (2001). Cardiotoxicity with modern local anaesthetics: is there a safer choice? *Drugs,* Vol.61, pp.333-342.

Mcleod G.A., Munishankar B., & Columb M.O. (2007). An isobolographic analysis of diamorphine and levobupivacaine for epidural analgesia in early labour. *British Journal of Anaesthesia,* Vol.98, pp.497-502.

O'Meara M.E., & Gin T. (1993). Comparison of 0.125% bupivacaine with 0.125% bupivacaine and clonidine as extradural analgesia in the first stage of labour. *British Journal of Anaesthesia,* Vol.71, pp.651-656.

Paech M.J., Pavy T.J., Orlikowski C.E., & Evans S.F. (2000). Patient-controlled epidural analgesia in labor: the addition of clonidine to bupivacaine-fentanyl. *Regional Anesthesia and Pain Medicine,* Vol.25, pp.34-40.

Page J.P., Bonnin M., Bolandard F., Vernis L., Lavergne B., Baud O., Bazin J.E., & Vendittelli F. (2008). [Epidural analgesia in obstetrics: anaesthesiologists practice in Auvergne]. *Annales Françaises d'Anesthésie et de Réanimation,* Vol.27, pp.685-693.

Parker R.K., Connelly N.R., Lucas T., Serban S., Pristas R., Berman E., & Gibson C. (2007). Epidural clonidine added to a bupivacaine infusion increases analgesic duration in labor without adverse maternal or fetal effects. *Journal of Anesthesia,* Vol.21, pp.142-147.

Polley L.S., Columb M.O., Naughton N.N., Wagner D.S., van de Ven C.J., & Goralski K.H. (2003). Relative analgesic potencies of levobupivacaine and ropivacaine for epidural analgesia in labor. *Anesthesiology,* Vol.99, pp.1354-1358.

Polley L.S., Columb M.O., Wagner D.S., & Naughton N.N. (1998). Dose-dependent reduction of the minimum local analgesic concentration of bupivacaine by sufentanil for epidural analgesia in labor. *Anesthesiology,* Vol.89, pp.626-632.

Powell H.C., Kalichman M.W., Garrett R.S., & Myers R.R. (1988). Selective vulnerability of unmyelinated fiber Schwann cells in nerves exposed to local anesthetics. *Laboratory Investigation,* Vol.59, pp.271-280.

Purdue Pharma. Chirocaine Injection. http://www.painhealth.com/medical-product X.asp?i=11516 . 2011.

Racle J.P., Benkhadra A., Poy J.Y., & Gleizal B. (1987). Prolongation of isobaric bupivacaine spinal anesthesia with epinephrine and clonidine for hip surgery in the elderly. *Anesthesia Analgesia,* Vol.66, pp.442-446.

Reid D. (1998). Differential nerve block. *Canadian Journal of Anaesthesia,* Vol.45, pp.1039-1043.

Robinson A.P., Lyons G.R., Wilson R.C., Gorton H.J., & Columb M.O. (2001). Levobupivacaine for epidural analgesia in labor: the sparing effect of epidural fentanyl. *Anesthesia Analgesia,* Vol.92, pp.410-414.

Roelants F., Lavand'homme P.M., & Mercier-Fuzier V. (2005). Epidural administration of neostigmine and clonidine to induce labor analgesia: evaluation of efficacy and local anesthetic-sparing effect. *Anesthesiology,* Vol.102, pp.1205-1210.

Sah N., Vallejo M., Phelps A., Finegold H., Mandell G., & Ramanathan S. (2007). Efficacy of ropivacaine, bupivacaine, and levobupivacaine for labor epidural analgesia. *Journal of Clinical Anesthesia,* Vol.19, pp.214-217.

Sautou V, Bonnin M, Bourdeau D, Bazin M, Tixier S, Dualé C, Chopineau J, Bazin JE. Etude pharmacologique de stabilité des poches pré-remplies de levobupivacaine avec adjonction de sufentanil et de clonidine. *Annales Françaises d'Anesthésie et de Réanimation.* 2011 (abstract).

Singelyn F.J., Gouverneur J.M., & Robert A. (1996). A minimum dose of clonidine added to mepivacaine prolongs the duration of anesthesia and analgesia after axillary brachial plexus block. *Anesthesia Analgesia,* Vol.83, pp.1046-1050.

Sufang G., Padmadas S.S., Fengmin Z., Brown J.J., & Stones R.W. (2007). Delivery settings and caesarean section rates in China. *Bulletin of the World Health Organization,* Vol.85, pp.755-762.

Tixier S., Bonnin M., Bolandard F., Vernis L., Lavergne B., Bazin J.E., & Dualé C. (2010). Continuous patient-controlled epidural infusion of levobupivacaine plus sufentanil in labouring primiparous women: effects of concentration. *Anaesthesia,* Vol.65, pp.573-580.

Tremlett M.R., Kelly P.J., Parkins J., Hughes D., & Redfern N. (1999). Low-dose clonidine infusion during labour. *British Journal of Anaesthesia,* Vol.83, pp.257-261.

Vernis L., Dualé C., Storme B., Mission J.P., Rol B., & Schoeffler P. (2004). Perispinal analgesia for labour followed by patient-controlled infusion with bupivacaine and sufentanil: combined spinal-epidural vs. epidural analgesia alone. *European Journal of Anaesthesiology,* Vol.21, pp.186-192.

Wallet F., Clement H.J., Bouret C., Lopez F., Broisin F., Pignal C., Schoeffler M., Derre E., Charpiat B., Huissoud C., Aubrun F., & Viale J.P. (2010). Effects of a continuous low-dose clonidine epidural regimen on pain, satisfaction and adverse events during labour: a randomized, double-blind, placebo-controlled trial. *European Journal of Anaesthesiology,* Vol.27, pp.441-447.

3

Patient-Controlled Analgesia After Major Abdominal Surgery in the Elderly Patient

Viorel Gherghina, Gheorghe Nicolae, Iulia Cindea,
Razvan Popescu and Catalin Grasa
*Emergency Clinical County Hospital Constanta,
Romania*

1. Introduction

Effective pain management of acute postoperative pain is mainly a humanitarian action that influences directly the length of recovery and hospitalization, therefore having important medical, economic, and social consequences.

As the complexity of analgesic therapies increases, priorities of care must be established to balance aggressive pain management with measures to prevent or minimize adverse events and to ensure high quality and safe care.

Analgesia remains the primary pharmacologic intervention for managing hospitalized surgical patients. Unintended advancing sedation and respiratory depression are two of the most serious analgesic-related adverse events. Multiple factors, including analgesic dose, route of administration, duration of therapy, patient-specific factors, and desired goals of therapy, can influence the occurrence of these adverse events. Furthermore, there is an urgent need to educate all members of the health care team about the dangers and potential attributes of administration of sedating medications concomitant with analgesia and the importance of initiating rational multimodal analgesic plans to help avoid adverse events.

Elderly patients frequently pose many challenges perioperatively that are not often seen in younger patients. Dementia, frailty, impaired ability to care for oneself, and malnourishment may be present at baseline and are likely to worsen postoperatively. The elderly are at increased risk of acute delirium and cognitive impairment postoperatively, which often complicates recovery and discharge placement.

Patient-controlled analgesia is a modern and effective method of postoperative pain management, mostly after major abdominal surgeries.

Using a special analgesia pump, the patient can self-administer the analgesic as needed, in pre-established bolus doses to which an analgesic basal infusion may not be associated.

Patient-controlled analgesia (PCA) with intravenous morphine and patient-controlled epidural analgesia with a local anaesthetic (sufentanyl-bupivacaine) in combination with an opioid (PCEA) are two new techniques, theoretically beneficial. However, these techniques have been inadequately evaluated in elderly people.

A relatively limited number of studies performed a comparative evaluation of the effects of various perioperative analgesic techniques on the overall recovery of elderly patients and therefore we undertook a prospective, randomized study to compare the effectiveness and possible adverse effects on postoperative pain and recovery of two analgesia and anesthesia techniques: general anesthesia in combination with epidural analgesia, followed postoperatively by PCEA (sufentanyl-bupivacaine), and general anesthesia followed postoperatively by PCA with morphine administered intravenously.

Secondly, we evaluated the mental status of patients after developing respiratory, hemodynamic, and gastrointestinal complications.

2. Background

One of the most common methods for providing postoperative analgesia is via patient-controlled analgesia (PCA). Although the typical approach is to administer opioids via a programmable infusion pump, other drugs and other modes of administration are available.

Patient-controlled analgesia (PCA) is commonly assumed to imply on-demand, intermittent, intravenous (IV) administration of opioids under patient control (with or without a continuous background infusion).

This technique is based on the use of a sophisticated microprocessor-controlled infusion pump that delivers a preprogrammed dose of opioid when the patient pushes a demand button. PCA is a conceptual framework for administration of analgesics . The broader concept of PCA is not restricted to a single class of analgesics or a single route or mode of administration. Nor should PCA imply the mandatory presence of a sophisticated and expensive infusion device. Any analgesic given by any route of delivery (i.e., oral, subcutaneous, epidural, peripheral nerve catheter, or transdermal) can be considered PCA if administered on immediate patient demand in sufficient quantities.

2.1 Historical perspective

Gross undertreatment of acute pain has been well chronicled over the last quarter century and likely continues today. The traditional approach of IM opioids given *pro re nata* (prn) results in at least 50% of patients experiencing inadequate pain relief after surgery.

Marks and Sachar's landmark 1973 publication ignited a philosophical revolution in practitioners' perception of the adequacy of conventional analgesic practices. Not only did this study document that a large proportion of hospitalized patients were undertreated, it also exposed that physicians and nurses are misinformed and lack sophistication regarding the effective use of opioid analgesics. This began the shift in intellectual milieu from the quest for the "perfect" analgesic (with an ever-expanding opioid pharmacopoeia) towards optimizing the mode of administration and delivery system for the (perfectly adequate) analgesic drugs that already existed.

Roe was the first to demonstrate, in 1963, that small IV doses of opioids provide more effective pain relief than conventional IM injections. Subsequently, Sechzer —the true pioneer of PCA—evaluated the analgesic response to small IV doses of opioid given on patient demand by a nurse in 1968 and then by machine in 1971 . Obviously, frequent administration of IV doses of opioid by nurses to large numbers of patients is impractical and cost prohibitive. Thus, the late 1960s witnessed development of PCA technologies.

In 1976, the first commercially available PCA pump, the "Cardiff Palliator," was developed at the Welsh National School of Medicine . Since then, PCA devices have evolved enormously in technological sophistication, ease of use, flexibility, and portability.

The smallest concentration at which pain was relieved was termed the "minimum effective analgesic concentration" (MEAC). Minimal analgesia is achieved with titration of opioid until the MEAC is achieved, which marks the difference between severe pain and analgesia. Furthermore, these investigators found a discrete concentration of opioid within an individual to consistently provide effective analgesia, whereas the discrete concentration that provided analgesia varied considerably among individuals, thus establishing that pharmacodynamic variability in response to opioids accounts for individual differences in dose requirements.

Pharmacokinetic variables (volume of distribution, rates of distribution and elimination) consistently failed to correlate with dose requirement; in contrast, an individual's hourly opioid dose and their plasma opioid concentration did correlate.

Two prerequisites for effective opioid analgesia were thus established:

1. individualize dosage and titrate to pain relief response to achieve the MEAC and establish analgesia,
2. maintain constant plasma opioid concentrations and avoid peaks and troughs .

These requirements cannot be achieved with prn or around-the-clock IM injections.

After titration to achieve the MEAC and establish analgesia, patients use PCA to maintain plasma opioid concentrations at or just above their individual MEAC ("optimal plasma concentration"). In contrast, patients receiving IM bolus injections experience significant periods of severe pain with their plasma opioid concentrations less than their individual MEAC, followed by periods of "overshoot" more than the optimal plasma concentration resulting in excessive sedation, possible respiratory depression, and no better pain relief.

2.2 PCA modes and dosing variables

PCA has several modes of administration. The two most common are demand dosing (a fixed-size dose is self-administered intermittently) and continuous infusion plus demand dosing (a constant-rate fixed background infusion is supplemented by patient demand dosing). Nearly all modern PCA devices offer both modes.

Less commonly available and less studied modes of administration include infusion demand (in which successful demands are administered as an infusion), preprogrammed variable-rate infusion plus demand dosing (in which the infusion rate is preprogrammed on an internal clock to vary or turn off altogether by time of day), and variable-rate feedback infusion plus demand dosing (in which a microprocessor monitors demands and controls the infusion rate accordingly).

For all modes of PCA, there are the following basic variables: initial loading dose, demand dose, lockout interval, background infusion rate, and 1-h and 4-h limits. The initial loading dose allows for titration of medication when activated by the programmer (not the patient).

The initial loading dose can be used by nurses in the postanesthesia care unit (PACU) to titrate opioid to the MEAC or by postsurgical nurses to give "breakthrough" doses.

The demand dose (sometimes called incremental or PCA dose) is the quantity of analgesic given to the patient on activation of the demand button. To prevent overdosage by continual demand, all PCA devices use a lockout interval (or delay), which is the length of time after a successful patient demand during which the device will not administer another demand dose (even if the patient pushes the demand button).

The background or continuous infusion is a constant rate infusion that is administered regardless of whether the patient activates demand doses. Some devices allow entry of 1-h and/or 4-h limits, with the intent of programming the device to limit the patient over either 1-h or 4-h intervals to less total cumulative dose than were they to successfully activate the demand button at the end of each lockout interval. Use of these 1-h and 4-h limits is controversial.

Proponents argue that these limits provide additional safety, whereas detractors argue that no data demonstrate enhanced safety. Moreover, if a patient uses enough demand doses to reach the 1-h or 4-h limit, they probably require more analgesic instead of being locked out from further access for the balance of the interval.

The alarm on most devices is nonspecific and nurses typically do not recognize if this condition has triggered the alarm. Most modern microprocessor-driven PCA devices allow for programming in the "PCA mode" (in which a continuous infusion is not offered) or the "PCA + continuous mode." Whereas earlier PCA devices allowed for entry of parameters in units of "mL" or "mg," many newer devices also allow for entry in "µg" units, thereby reducing the potential for programming error when using fentanyl or sufentanil.

The demand dose and lockout interval (as well as the background infusion—see the hazards of continuous background infusions with IV-PCA under the safety section below) deserve further discussion. In practice, most patients have an inherent maximum frequency of demands. Thus, if the demand dose is too small, they refrain from making demands and may become frustrated with PCA, resulting in poor pain relief .

For PCA to be successful, the demand dose should produce appreciable analgesia with a single demand . However, if the demand dose is too large, plasma drug concentration may eventually reach toxic levels. There is an optimal range of doses for each opioid, albeit a wide enough dose range to accommodate the pharmacodynamic variability in response to opioids among individuals.

It is possible to coach patients to increase the demand rate. If the demand dose is changed during PCA treatment, patients will alter their demand rate to accommodate the change, thus maintaining a consistent plasma opioid concentration.

The lockout interval is designed to prevent overdose. Ideally, it should be long enough for the patient to experience the maximal effect of one dose before another is permitted, thus preventing "stacking" of doses. Therefore, speed of onset of analgesia is paramount in setting the lockout interval. Based on this rationale, one might consider using a slightly shorter lockout interval when using the "fentanyl family of opioids" compared to morphine or hydromorphone.

However, once titration to MEAC has been achieved, there appears to be no clinically appreciable major differences in time of onset of analgesia among the opioids commonly used for PCA . The rate of drug distribution (flux) between plasma and brain is a useful concept in determining the lockout interval. While drug flux is positive, there is net movement of drug from plasma to brain and drug effect increases. The next dose should be administered when net flux becomes negative, i.e., when drug is leaving the brain and effect has peaked.

The change from positive to negative flux occurs over a similar length of time for diverse opioids. Many studies examined the relative brain and spinal cord central nervous system (CNS) concentration profiles of opioids. CNS concentration was expressed as a percentage of its maximum value. Relative onset was defined as the time that the relative CNS concentration first reached 80% of maximum and relative duration was defined as the period during which the concentration remained more than 80%. For an IV bolus dose of all the common opioids, relative onset varies from approximately 1 min for alfentanil to 6 min for morphine, and relative durations are 2 min and 96 min, respectively.

They concluded that, although all of the common opioids (except alfentanil) have kinetic and dynamic properties suitable for IV-PCA, the relatively long duration of morphine makes it particularly suited for a gradual titration approach.

Furthermore, titration is improved by frequent administration of small doses after the initial "loading" period. Thus, there appears to be pharmacokinetic rationale for the empirically derived use of 5–12 min lockout intervals for the opioids commonly used for IV-PCA.

2.3 Choice of analgesic

All of the common opioids have been used successfully for IV-PCA, with morphine having been studied the most. Whichever opioid is chosen for IV-PCA, knowledge of its pharmacology is prerequisite for setting the dosing variables of the PCA device. A review of the practical clinical pharmacology of opioids, as it pertains to management of IV-PCA, is essential.

Parenteral opioids have three profiles of μ opiate-receptor binding capacity: pure agonists, agonist-antagonists, and partial agonists. Pure agonists are mainstays of acute pain management because they provide full μ-receptor binding, i.e., there is no analgesic ceiling (e.g., titration of more opioid results in better pain relief).

There is a "clinical ceiling" in that side effects such as sedation, specifically respiratory depression, often prevent further dosing before achieving adequate pain relief. The μ agonists are equally effective at equianalgesic doses (e.g., 10 mg of morphine = 2 mg of hydromorphone = 100 mg of meperidine). Similarly, there are no differences in side-effect profile, although individual patients may experience reproducible nausea and vomiting or pruritus with one drug but not another.

All μ-agonists reduce propulsive gut activity and coordination, contributing to postoperative ileus. Contrary to surgical myth, no individual μ-agonist has less effect on gut motility: in conventional IV-PCA doses, morphine, meperidine, and fentanyl have similar effects on the bile ducts and sphincter of Oddi.

There is evidence that agonist-antagonists share this activity to a lesser degree. Metabolites and routes of elimination differ markedly between μ-agonists, providing one rationale for choosing an opioid for IV-PCA.

The agonist-antagonist opioids provide κ-receptor activation and μ-receptor antagonism. Although they are marketed as having a ceiling effect on respiratory depression, thereby providing a greater margin of safety, this effect appears only at very large doses relative to μ-agonists. Most importantly, the agonist-antagonists possess an analgesic ceiling, rendering them unable to reliably provide a level of pain relief comparable to the μ-agonists. Thus, although the successful use of an agonist-antagonist for IV-PCA has been described for gynecologic surgery , they are not commonly used in clinical practice and would not reliably provide adequate analgesia for moderate-to-severe pain conditions.

Furthermore, agonist-antagonists can provoke an acute withdrawal response in patients who have already received a μ-agonist or are maintained on one chronically. As a result of ς-receptor activation, they also have a frequent incidence of disturbing psychotomimetic side effects.

Interestingly, there appears to be a major gender difference in response to agonist-antagonists. Although women consistently experience dose-dependent analgesia, an antianalgesic response with increased pain compared with placebo was observed in men receiving nalbuphine . Partial agonists produce only a partial response in binding to μ receptors, thereby limiting the analgesia that can be achieved. They are not used commonly for IV-PCA.

Morphine remains the "gold standard" for IV-PCA, as the most studied and most commonly used IV-PCA drug. It is important to note that morphine has an active metabolite—morphine-6-glucuronide (M6G)—that also produces analgesia, sedation, and respiratory depression. Whereas morphine is eliminated mainly by glucuronidation, its active metabolite relies predominantly on renal excretion for elimination. Prolonged and profound delayed onset respiratory depression has been reported in patients with renal failure receiving parenteral morphine.

Hydromorphone is a good alternative for morphine-intolerant patients or those with altered renal function because it is metabolized primarily in the liver and excreted primarily as an inactive glucuronide metabolite .A demand dose of 0.2 mg of Hydromorphine is considered equi-analgesic to 1.0 mg of morphine since it is approximately six times as potent as morphine.Following this analgesic advantage over morphine, it is commonly used PCApumps at a concentration of 0.5 mg/ml or 1 mg/ml. Hydromorphine is ideally suited for opioid-tolerant patients, increasing the interval between refilling the drug reservoir.

Fentanyl is considered 80–100 times as potent as morphine with single doses or brief periods of administration. However, because of its short duration of action, particularly in the early phase of administration (owing to redistribution pharmacokinetics), double-blind IV-PCA comparator trials have suggested 25–30 μg fentanyl to be equianalgesic to 1 mg morphine as an IV-PCA demand dose, i.e., 33–40 times as potent as morphine. Fentanyl has a quicker onset than morphine and better suited for iv-PCA probably due its lipophilicity. Fentanyl has been used successfully for IV-PCA . It is an excellent alternative for morphine-intolerant patients and is suitable for patients with renal failure because it does not rely on renal excretion for elimination.

Although meperidine has traditionally been the second most common µ-agonist opioid prescribed for IV-PCA, its routine use for IV-PCA is strongly discouraged . Meperidine has a neurotoxic metabolite, normeperidine, that possesses no analgesic property and relies mostly on renal excretion for elimination. Normeperidine accumulation causes CNS excitation, resulting in a range of toxic reactions from anxiety and tremors to grand mal seizures. Unwitnessed seizures with loss of airway reflexes can result in severe permanent anoxic brain injury or death.

Use of sufentanil, alfentanil, and remifentanil for IV-PCA has been reported, with sufentanil studied the most . With sufentanil, an initial demand dose of 4–6 µg appears to be most appropriate. In contrast to the longer-acting opioids discussed above, a small background infusion may be necessary to sustain analgesia with sufentanil. Owen et al. could not identify an optimal dose and administration rate for alfentanil, concluding that it is not a useful drug for IV-PCA. Because of its ultra-short duration, remifentanil is probably only appropriate for IV-PCA use in short duration, severe episodic pain conditions such as labor pain.

3. Materials and method

This prospective, randomized study was approved by the Ethics Committee of the Emergency Clinical Hospital Constanta and included 70 patients undergoing major elective abdominal surgery.

The patient inclusion criteria in the study were: over 70 years old; status ASA I -III; scheduled major abdominal surgery; normal preoperative mental status, defined by score≥ 8 in the adapted Abbreviated Mental Test (AMT–Table 1); absence of contraindications for epidural anesthesia (clinical or laboratory); absence of extreme malnutrition or of cerebral vascular insufficiency.

Age
Time
Hospital address
Year
Hospital name
Recognizes two persons (for example, physician, assistant)
Date of birth
Year First World War began
Name of the President of the country
Counts backwards from 20 to 1

*The patients were asked to answer these 10 questions.Each correct answer received one point.

Table 1. Abbreviated Mental Test (AMT)*

On the day preceding surgery, during the pre-anesthesia interview, the patients signed the informed consent and received written and verbal instruction regarding the use of PCA or PCEA.

The patients were randomly assigned to two groups, using the random numbers list method: the PCA group - 35 patients with intravenous postoperative analgesia (morphine), the PCEA group - 35 patients with postoperative analgesia by epidural catheter (sufentanyl-bupivacaine).

In the PCEA group, before surgery, a thoracic (T7 - T11) epidural catheter was inserted in each patient, depending on the location of the surgery.

All surgeries were performed under balanced general anesthesia (induction with propofol, sufentanyl and atracurium, maintenance with sevoflurane, sufentanyl and atracurium) with standard intraoperative monitoring. After surgery, the patients were transferred to the Postoperative Care Unit.

In the PCA group, analgesia was initiated with a loading dose of 5 mg morphine intravenously, and subsequently the PCA analgesic pump (B.Braun Melsungen) was programmed to provide 1.5 mg morphine boluses intravenously with a blocking interval of 8 minutes.

For the postoperative analgesia in the PCEA group, we used a combination of bupivacaine 0.125% and sufentanyl 5 µg/ml administered by the patient-controlled analgesia pump (B.Braun Melsungen). The settings of the pump parametrs were: 2-3 ml bolus, safety interval of 12 minutes, and a basal infusion rate of 3 - 5 ml/hour.

In order to quantify the severity of postoperative pain, the patients were asked to use the 10 cm Visual Analogue Scale (VAS) graded from 0 cm (no pain) to 10 cm (unbearable pain). The VAS score was recorded daily at rest after coughing at 8 am, 12 pm, 8 pm, during the first 5 days after surgery. To optimize analgesia and minimize sedation and haemodynamic instability, the patient control setting was checked throughout the day for individual adjuatments.

When inadequate analgesia was noted (VAS>3), additiona injectable acetaminophen (1 g i.v.) or ketoprofen (100 mg i.v.) was administered.

Overall, the patient satisfaction score regarding postoperative analgesia was recorded on the 5th day after surgery (insufficient analgesia = 0, relatively good analgesia =1, good analgesia=2, excellent =3).

The patients' sedation was evaluated using a 4-point sedation scale (0=awake, opens eyes spontaneously, 1 = slightly sleepy, openes eyes on verbal stimuli, 2=moderately sleepy, opens eyes on tactile stimuli, nociceptive, 3=exremely sleepy, unresponsive).

The incidence of adverse effects caused by the opioid was evaluated: pruritus (present or absent), nausea or vomiting (present or absent).

These parametrs were recorded daily at 8 am, 12 pm, 8 pm, during the first 5 days after surgery.

The sensitive block was tested daily using the blunt pin prick technique as well as the motor block using the Bromage scale (0= free movement of the lower limb,1= cannot lift the extended lower limb; 2= cannot flex the knee, 3= lower limb completely motionless).

The blood pressure, heart rate, respiration rate, SpO2, were monitored every two hours during the first 5 days after surgery.

Gastrointestinal function was evaluated by systematically questioning the patients regarding the recovery of the digestive tolerance and transit of gases.

The statistical data proccessing was performed using the Student's t-tests and chi-square test. Values of <0.05 were considered statistically significant.

4. Results

A total number of 108 patients were scheduled for major abdominal surgical interventions at the Emergency Country Clinical Hospital in Constanta during this study.

Out of these, 38 (35%) were not included in the study for various reasons: patient (4%), severe cardiopulmonary conditions or MT score <8 (24%), neurological dysfunction (2%), patient death (6%).

The remaining 70 patients were randomly assigned to two groups: the PCA group, PCEA group.

Six patients did not complete the postoperative study or were excluded from the postoperative data analysis due to the absence of surgical resection (2 patients in each group) or to their non-compliance to the patient-controlled analgesia devices; these patients requested conventional analgesia (2 patients in the PCEA group).

Demographic and intraoperative data were comparable in both groups, and there were no statistically significant differences regarding the duration or type of surgery (Table 2).

No significant differences were noticed between the two groups regarding the intraoperative need for infusion solutions.

The patients in the PCEA group received less sevoflurane (p=0.0001) and sufentanyl intravenously (p=0.0001) during surgery, however they required significantly more ephedrine (p=0.0001) than the patients in the PCA group.

At the end of surgery, the duration of mechanical ventilation was similar in both groups, however extubation was performed significantly earlier in the PCEA group than in the PCA group.

The duration of patient-controlled analgesia was similar in both groups (PCA GROUP -70 ± 22 hours), avalid situation concerning the daily number of analgesic boluses used by the patients. The postoperative patient-controlled analgesic consumption is presented in Table 3.

The VAS score analysis shows that PCEA ensured significantly better (p=0.0001) postoperative pain management than PCA at rest (PCEA 22.93 ± 10, PCA 38.74 ± 8) and after coughing (PCEA 32.45 ± 13.05, PCA 45.40 ± 11.6) during the first 5 days after surgery .

During the first day after surgery, a significantly smaller number of patients in the PCEA group requested additional analgesia (VAS ≥4) compared with the patients in the PCA group (Table 4).

Parameter	PCA group (n=35)	PCEA group (n=35)
Age (years)	76.8 ± 4.7	± 5.6
Weight (kg)	69.3 ± 15.5	66.5 ±14.2
Gender	17 F/18M	15 F/20M
Surgery		
Colectomy	26 (74%)	20 (57%)
Gastrectomy	2 (6%)	6 (17%)
Cephalic pancreatectomy	5 (14%)	7 (20%)
Absence of resection	2 (6%)	2 (6 %)
Mean duration of surgery (minutes) (range)	242 (172 -295)	230 (180-305)
Average sevoflurane (%)	0.8 (0.6 – 1)	0.5 (0.4-0.6)*
Sufentanyl intravenously (μg/kg)	1.7 (1.3-2.2)	0.3 (0.3-0.4)
Crystalloids (l)	5 (4-6)	5 (4-6)
Colloids (l)	0.5 (0-1)	1.0 (0.5-1.5)
Incidence of systolic hypotension intraoperatively (<90 mmHg)	21 (60%)	26 (74%)
Duration of systolic hypotension intraoperatively (minutes)	5 (0 -209	15 ((5-30)
Ephedrine intravenously (mg)	0 (0-0)	12 (6 -36%)*
Postoperative extubation (minutes)	60 (32-90)	30 (17 -57)*
Duration of postoperative mechanical ventilation (minutes)	27 (10-65)	27 (12-45)

Data presented as median ± DS, median or numeric
*p< 0.05 between the two treatment groups

Table 2. Demographic and perioperative data of study groups

Postoperative day	Morphine sulphate i.v. (mg/day) PCA group	Bupivacaine epidural (mg/day) PCEA group	Epidural sufentanyl (μg/day) PCEA group
1	25 (24 - 44)	169 (150-236)	68 (57-94.5)
2	19 (8 -32)	158 (120-216)	63 (48-87)
3	10 (0 -21)	127 (94-153)	51 (37-61)
4	0 (0-0)	50 (0 -120)	20 (0 -48)
5	0 (0-0)	0 (0-0)	0 (-0)

Data presented as median;
PCA group = intravenous patient-controlled analgesia
PCEA group = epidural patient-controlled analgesia

Table 3. Postoperative consumption of patient –controlled analgesic

Postoperative day	Number of patient who required acetaminophen intravenously		Number of patient who required ketoprofen intravenously	
	PCAgroup no.(%)	PCEA group no.(%)	PCAgroup no.(%)	PCEA group no.(%)
1	18 (54)	11(35)	15 (45)	5 (16)*
2	18 (54)	15 (48)	6 (18)	3 (10)
3	19 (58)	17 (55)	3 (9)	3 (10)
4	15 (45)	17 (55)	2 (6)	3 (10)
5	12 (36)	10 (32)	1 (3)	0 (0)

Data presented as n.(%) *$p<0.05$ between the two study groups; The PCA group = intravenous patient-controlled analgesia; The PCEA group = epidural patient-controlled analgesia

Table 4. Postoperative consumption of additionally requested analgesic in the two study groups

The patient satisfaction score was significantly higher ($p=0.012$) in the PCEA group compared to the PCA group (Table 5).

Parameter	PCA group (n=33)	PCEA group (n= 33)
Recovery of intestinal transit (hours)	115 (90-144)	80 (60 -120)*
Digestive tolerance (hours)	182 (140-240)	142 (120 -164)*
Nausea and vomiting	10 (30%)	10 (32%)
Systolic arterial hypotension (<90 mmHg)	0 (0%)	5 (16%)
SpO2 <95%	5 (15%)	3 (10%)
Moderate pulmonary complications	2 (6%)	3 (10%)
Major pulmonary complications	1 (3%)	1 (3%)
Urinary tract infections	5 (15%)	1 (3%)
Pruritus	1 (3%)	1 (3%)
Postoperative delirium	8 (24%)	8 (26%)
Duration of hospitalization (days)	11.5 (8 -16)	10.5 (8-15)
Patients satisfaction score (no. of patients with score 0/1/2/3)	0/3/19/11	0/1/9/21*
AMT score (no. of patients with score < 8/9/10)	5/13/15	1/7/23

Data presented as n.(%);
*$p<0.05$ between the two study groups;
The PCA group = intravenous patient-controlled analgesia;
The PCEA group = epidural patient-controlled analgesia;
Patient satisfaction score is: insufficient =0, relatively good= 1, good= 2, excellent =3

Table 5. Postoperative status, adverse events, and patient satisfaction score in the two study groups

The daily recorder AMT scores had, before surgery, similar values in both groups, while after surgery the PCA group had lower values during the 4th and 5th day after surgery.

There were no significant differences between the two groups regarding the daily values of oxygenation during the first 5 days after surgery and the number of minor occurrences of asymptomatic hypoxia detected by pulse oximetry. Three patients in the PCA group and 2 patients in the PCEA group had at least one episode of a fall in the SpO2 to between 90 and 95%. One patient had a much lower SpO2 value between 85 and 90%.

Five patients in the PCEA group had postoperative hypotension corrected by volume repletion. This event was not noted in the PCA group.

The frequency of postoperative delirium was similar in the PCA group (8 patients, 24%) and the PCEA group (8 patients, 26%). The patients with delirium did not have an analgesic consumption or pain score different from those without delirium.

Postoperatively, the AMT score was lower in the PCA group compared to the PCEA group.

Recovery of digestive tolerance (p=0.019) and bowel movement (p= 0.005) occured significantly sooner in the PCA group compared to the PCEA group.

The incidence of pruritus, nausea and vomiting was almost equal in the two study groups.

The duration of hospitalization was similar for the patients in the two groups (Table 5).

5. Discussion

Effective analgesia reduces perioperative stress and the rate of complications, extremely important issues in abdominal surgery. The particularities of the elderly patient require ongoing efforts to adapt current analgesic techniques in order to improve the prognosis of surgeries in this category of patients.

The main conclusion of our study is that in elderly patients , patient-controlled analgesia techniques, intravenously or epidurally, ensure an efficient management of postoperative pain.

Epidural analgesia provides better control of postoperative pain at rest as well as after coughing, without increasing the incidence of complications, a compared to intravenous analgesia. Improved mental status of the patients and faster recovery of the digestive function were noted in the PCEA group.

In elderly patients, the difficulties associated with the use of patient-controlled analgesia techniques were mainly caused by the inability to lean the correct use of analgesic pumps.

Previous studies revealed the need for a closer supervision of elderly patients and the compulsory frequent adjustment of the administered doses, however, in our study the adjustment of the initial settings of patient-controlled analgesia was seldom necessary. In the PCA group, the initial setting was not changed because no signs of overdose were recorded, and in the PCEA group only 5 patients (16%) required alterations of the bolus dosages, to adapt it to the patient requirements.

Learning and acquiring the concept of patient control obviously involves an adequate preoperative mental status. The preoperative patient selection using the AMT scores enabled us to identify those with pre-existing cognitive impairments and consequently these patients were not enrolled in the study .This aspect might explain why only 3 % of the selected patients refused the patient-controlled devices and requested conventional analgesia. The high level of acceptance by the selected patients encourages us to recommend the routine pre-operative use of the AMT to ensure effective management of postoperative care in elderly patients .

The analysis of the patient satisfaction scores reveals the superiority of the PCEA techniques, explained by the better analgesic efficiency associated to the low incidence of adverse events. An important issue to consider is that in the PCEA mode patient control is partial, since it is possible to establish a basal analgesic perfusion rate. This aspect is extremely important for confused or sleepy patients who cannot control effectively the analgesic device. The intravenous continuous analgesic infusion is not recommended since it involves a higher risk of respiratory depression even at low doses .

Abdominal epidural analgesia improves the postoperative recovery of the intestinal transit compared to parenteral analgesia. In our study, recovery of bowel movement and digestive tolerance in the PCA group were delayed, compared to the PCEA group. Clinical studies in which the epidural catheter was located at T12 or lower did not show any benefits regarding the recovery of the intestinal function , that is why we took care to always place the cather at the thoracic level.

The incidence of pulmonary complications in this study was similar to that noted in other studies with younger patients undergoing the same type of surgeries. The choice of analgesic techniques does not seem to have any influence on the incidence of moderate or major pulmonary complications.

The cardiovascular changes were clinically insignificant. As expected, in the PCEA group the hemodynamic instability was higher intraoperatively, requiring a higher consumption of ephedrine, or postoperatively, when 5 patients experienced episodes of moderate hypotension.

In the patients of the PCEA group, the risk of orthostatic hypotension and motor blockage of the lower limbs during postoperative mobilization may neutralize the benefit of faster postoperative recovery. In our study, the adjustment of pre-established analgesic doses may explain the lack of the significant hemodynamic instability or motor blockage.

6. Conclusion

This study shows that patient-controlled analgesic techniques, regardless of the epidural or parental route used, are effective in elderly patients.

An epidural analgesia is better than parenteral analgesia and ensures better pain management with improved mental status and faster recovery of intestinal activity, without influencing cardiorespiratory morbidity.

This postoperative analgesia method is a new, promising technique for elderly patients undergoing major surgery.

7. References

Agnelli, G. (2004). Prevention of venous thromboembolism in surgical patients. *Circulation*, Vol. 110, No. 24, Suppl. IV, (December 2004), pp. 4-12, ISSN: 1524-4539

Bartha, E.; Carlsson, P. & Kalman, S. (2006). Evaluation of costs and effects of epidural analgesia and patient-controlled intravenous analgesia after major abdominal surgery. *British Journal of Anaesthesia*, Vol. 96, No. 1, (January 2006), pp. 111-117, ISSN 1471-6771

Bauer, A. & Boeckxstaens, G. (2004). Mechanisms of postoperative ileus. *Neurogastroenterology & Motility*, Vol. 16, Issue Supplement s2, (October 2004), pp. 54-60

Beilin, B.; Shavit, Y. & Trabekin, E. (2003). The effects of postoperative pain management on immune response to surgery. *Anesthesia & Analgesia*, Vol. 97, No. 3, (September 2003), pp. 822-827, ISSN 1526-7598

Bombeli, T. & Spahn, D. (2004). Updates in perioperative coagulation: Physiology and management of thromboembolism and haemorrhage. *British Journal of Anaesthesia*, Vol. 93, No. 2, (August 2004), pp. 275-287, ISSN 1471-6771

Devereaux, P.; Goldman, L. & Cook, D. (2005). Perioperative cardiac events in patients undergoing noncardiac surgery: A review of the magnitude of the problem, the pathophysiology of the events and methods to estimate and communicate risk. *Canadian Medical Association Journal*, Vol. 173, No. 6, (September 2005), pp. 627-634, ISSN 1488-2329

Fong, H.; Sands, L. & Leung, J. (2006). The role of postoperative analgesia in delirium and cognitive decline in elderly patients: A systematic review. *Anesthesia & Analgesia*, Vol. 102, No. 4, (April 2006), pp. 1255-1266, ISSN 1526-7598

Groeben, H.; Schäfer, B. & Pavlakovic, G. (2002). Lung function under high thoracic segmental epidural anesthesia with ropivacaine or bupivacaine in patients with severe obstructive pulmonary disease undergoing breast surgery. *Anesthesiology*, Vol. 96, No. 3, (March 2002), pp. 536-541, ISSN 0003-3022

Holte, K. & Kehlet, H. (2002). Epidural anaesthesia and analgesia - effects on surgical stress responses and implications for postoperative nutrition. *Clinical Nutrition*, Vol. 21, No. 3, (June 2002), pp. 199-206, ISSN 0261-5614

Jørgensen, H.; Wetterslev, J. & Møiniche, S. (2000). Epidural local anaesthetics versus opioid-based analgesic regimens on postoperative gastrointestinal paralysis, PONV and pain after abdominal surgery. In: *Cochrane Database of Systematic Reviews 2001*, 23.10.2000, Available from http://www2.cochrane.org/reviews/en/ab001893.html

Kehlet, H. (1994). Postoperative pain relief—what is the issue? *British Journal of Anaesthesia*, Vol. 72, No. 4, (April 1994), pp. 375-378, ISSN 1471-6771

Kehlet, H. (1997). Multimodal approach to control postoperative pathophysiology and rehabilitation. *British Journal of Anaesthesia*, Vol. 78, No. 5, (May 1997), pp. 606-617, ISSN 1471-6771

Kehlet, H. & Holte, K. (2001). Effect of postoperative analgesia on surgical outcome. *British Journal of Anaesthesia*, Vol. 87, No. 1, (June 2001), pp. 62-72, ISSN 1471-6771

Kehlet, H. & Dahl, J. (2003). Anaesthesia, surgery and challenges in postoperative recovery. *The Lancet*, Vol. 362, No. 9399, (December 2003), pp. 1921-1928

Kehlet, H. (2008). Fast-track colorectal surgery. *The Lancet*, Vol. 371, No. 9615, (March 2008), pp. 791-793

Kehlet, H. & Wilmore, D. (2008). Evidence-based surgical care and the evolution of fast-track surgery. *Annals of Surgery*, Vol. 248, No. 2, (August 2008), pp. 189-198, ISSN 1528-1140

McLeod, G.; Davies, H. & Munnoch N. (2001). Postoperative pain relief using thoracic epidural analgesia: Outstanding success and disappointing failures. *Anaesthesia*, Vol. 56, No. 1, (January 2001), pp. 75-81

Moraca, R.; Sheldon, D. & Thirlby, R. (2003). The role of epidural anesthesia and analgesia in surgical practice. *Annals of Surgery*, Vol. 238, No. 5, (November 2003), pp. 663-673, ISSN 1528-1140

Mythen, M. (2005). Postoperative gastrointestinal tract dysfunction. *Anesthesia & Analgesia*, Vol. 100, No. 1, (January 2005), pp. 196-204, ISSN 1526-7598

Park, W.; Thompson, J. & Lee, K. (2001). Effect of epidural anesthesia and analgesia on perioperative outcome: A randomized, controlled veterans affairs cooperative study. *Annals of Surgery*, Vol. 234, No. 4, (October 2001), pp. 560-571, ISSN 1528-1140

Paulsen, E.; Porter, M. & Helmer, S. (2001). Thoracic epidural versus patient-controlled analgesia in elective bowel resections. *The American Journal of Surgery*, Vol. 182, No. 6, (December 2001), pp. 570-577, ISSN 0002-9610

Peyton, P.; Myles, P. & Silbert, B. (2003). Perioperative epidural analgesia and outcome after major abdominal surgery in high-risk patients. *Anesthesia & Analgesia*, Vol. 96, No. 2, (February 2003), pp. 548-554, ISSN 1526-7598

Pöpping, D.; Elia, N. & Marret, E. (2008). Protective effects of epidural analgesia on pulmonary complications after abdominal and thoracic surgery. *Archives of Surgery*, Vol. 143, No. 10, (October 2008), pp. 990-999

Rigg, J.; Jamrozik, K. & Myles, P. (2000). Design of the multicenter Australian study of epidural anesthesia and analgesia in major surgery: The MASTER trial. *Controlled Clinical Trials*, Vol. 21, No. 3, (June 2000), pp. 244-256

Rigg, J.; Jamrozik, K. & Myles, P. (2002). Epidural anaesthesia and analgesia an outcome of major surgery: A randomized trial. *The Lancet*, Vol. 359, No. 9314, (April 2002), pp. 1276-1282

Waurick, R. & Van Aken, H. (2005). Update in thoracic epidural anaesthesia. *Best Practice & Research: Clinical Anaesthesiology*, Vol. 19, No. 2, (June 2005), pp.201-213, ISSN 1521-6896

Werawatganon, T. & Charuluxananan, S. (2005). Patient controlled intravenous opioid analgesia versus continuous epidural analgesia for pain after intra-abdominal surgery. *Anesthesia & Analgesia*, Vol. 100, No. 5, (May 2005), pp. 1536, ISSN 1526-7598

Wheatley, R.; Shug, S. & Watson, D. (2001). Safety and efficacy of postoperative epidural analgesia. *British Journal of Anaesthesia*, Vol. 87, No. 1, (June 2001), pp. 47-61, ISSN 1471-6771

4

Epidural Analgesia for Perioperative Upper Abdominal Surgery

Arunotai Siriussawakul[1] and Aticha Suwanpratheep[2]
[1]*Department of Anesthesiology, Faculty of Medicine, Siriraj Hospital, Mahidol University, Bangkok,*
[2]*Division of Anesthesiology, Suratthani Hospital, Thailand*

1. Introduction

Uncontrolled postoperative pain and the pathophysiologic response to surgery following upper abdominal surgery may cause significant complications of many organ systems. Perioperative thoracic epidural analgesia (TEA), especially with a local anesthetic-based analgesic solution, can decrease the incidence of postoperative morbidity and mortality. In the case of the cardiovascular system, TEA may decrease the incidence of postoperative myocardial infarction by providing a favorable redistribution of coronary blood flow, attenuating the stress response, hypercoagulability and postoperative pain. As for the respiratory system, TEA provides superior analgesia, allowing patients to do deep breathing exercises and early ambulation. In a recent cohort study of 541 patients with chronic obstructive pulmonary disease, it was reported that TEA offered a preventive effect for postoperative pneumonia and a decrease in 30-day mortality. Stress-induced sympathetic outflow causes ileus and prolonged hospital stay. (van Lier et al., 2011) TEA can facilitate the return of gastrointestinal motility without contributing to anastomotic bowel dehiscence. Finally, TEA improves postoperative analgesia, resulting in increased patient satisfaction. (Hurley & Wu, 2009)

Although TEA provides many benefits, this technique has significant risks, including medication-related complications, epidural catheter-related complications and other complications associated with continuous epidural analgesia. This chapter will cover the practical aspects of thoracic epidural analgesia for perioperative upper abdominal surgery, including the anatomy of the thoracic epidural space, the technique of epidural block, drugs used for intraoperative and postoperative analgesia, and intraoperative and postoperative complications.

2. Approaches to the epidural space

Patients undergoing upper abdominal operations (cholecystectomy, esophagectomy, gastrectomy, hepatectomy and Whipple's operation) that involve large surgical incisions are suited for thoracic epidural anesthesia and analgesia. The recommended sites for epidural needle and catheter placement are at T6-8 levels. Catheter-incision-congruent epidural analgesia provides effective analgesia and minimizes side effects.

Standard monitors, including non-invasive blood pressure, pulse oximetry and electrocardiogram, should be applied before or after the positioning. Either the sitting or lateral decubitus position can be used. Exaggerated spinal flexion serves little benefit because thoracic facet joints primarily allow axial rotation. (Neal, 2004) Intravenous sedation (small doses of midazolam and fentanyl) for alleviating anxiety and supplemental oxygen should be given. The assistant should help the patient to hold the position during the entire procedure.

Identification of a specific vertebral interspace is generally based on palpitation at the surface landmarks of the spine. A line drawn between the inferior angles of the scapulae identifies the T7 spinous process (Fig. 1). The interspace can also be located by ultrasound imaging. This new technique has been reported useful for guiding neuraxial anesthetics in patients with prior instrumentation, and in obese and elderly patients. (Grey, 2010)

Since the midthoracic spinous processes are acutely angulated and the laminae become more vertically oriented as one progresses caudally (Fig 2), performing a paramedian approach is easier than a midline approach. The needle entry point is marked just off midline to avoid the process (Fig 1). The epidural space is commonly identified using a loss of resistance to air or the saline technique. An epidural catheter is advanced through the needle and 3 to 5 cm into the epidural space.

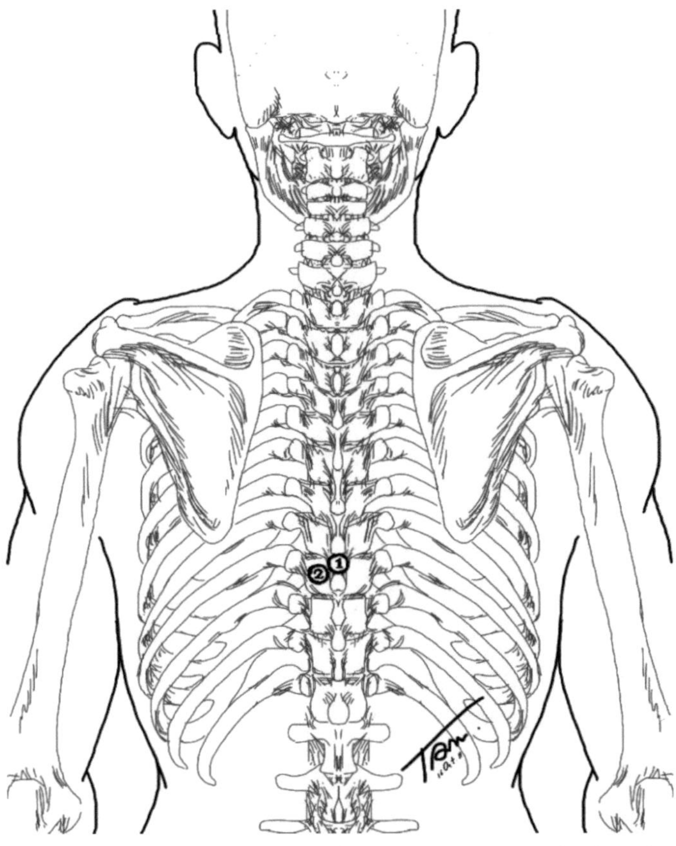

Fig. 1. Puncture sites at the surface landmark of the T7 level are at the line drawn between inferior angles of the scapulae: (1) median approach and (2) paramedian approach.

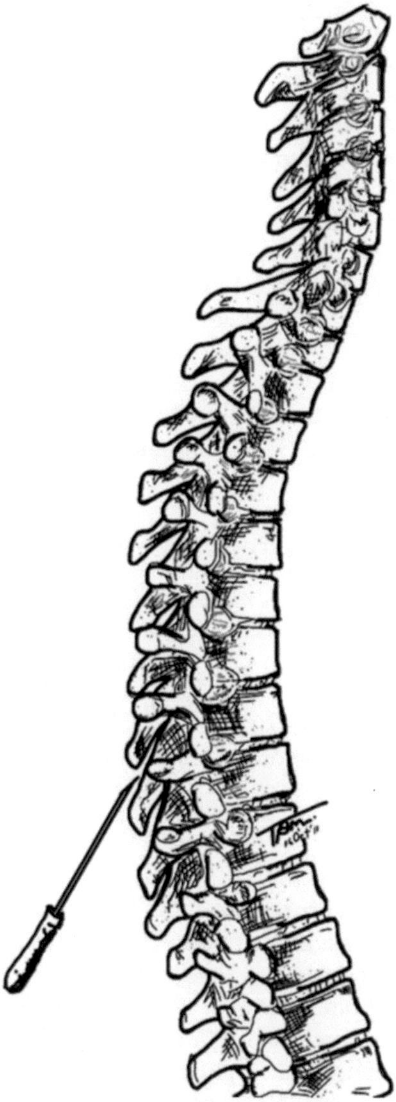

Fig. 2. Anatomy of thoracic spine: the spinous processes of the midthoracic spine have a very caudal angle. The acute insertion in the T7 level should be noted.

3. Epidural test dose

Once the catheter is placed, it is aspirated for the presence of blood or cerebrospinal fluid (CSF). A test dose of 60 mg of lidocaine and 1:200,000 of epinephrine is used to detect misplacement in the intrathecal or intravascular space. An intravenous injection of 15 μg of epinephrine typically produces an average heart rate increase of 30 beats per minute between 20 and 40 seconds after its administration. (Moore & Batra, 1981) A survey of academic medical centers in the United States found that 83% of the respondents indicated they use a test dose, whereas 6% do not. (Minzter et al., 2002)

4. Drugs used for intraoperative and postoperative analgesia

Several analgesics have been successfully used to provide optimal pain control via the thoracic epidural route. Because of their synergistic effects, combinations of low concentration local anesthetics (LA) with opioids are now standard· (Conacher &Slinger, 2003) The choice of LA for continuous epidural infusion varies. Lidocaine is the prototypical LA and is used epidurally in 1.5% to 2% concentrations. However, continuous infusion of lidocaine produces a tachyphylaxis phenomenon and increases the risk of LA toxicity. Bupivacaine remains the most commonly used LA and is commercially available as a racemic mixture of S(-) and R(+) enantiomers, but evidence suggests the R(+) enantiomer has greater cardiotoxicity. Pure S(-) enantiomer levobupivacaine has been developed for a potentially lower cardiotoxic profile. Both drugs provide comparable sensory block features, intraoperative hemodynamics and postoperative analgesia. (Cok et al., 2011) Commercial preparations of levobupivacaine have a 0.563% concentration of the molecule versus 0.5% in bupivacaine. Ropivacaine is another pure S(-) enantiomer that has been shown to be less cardiotoxic than bupivacaine.

Local Anesthetics	Concentration	Two-dermatome regression(min)
Lidocaine	1.5 - 2%	60 - 100
Bupivacaine	0.5 – 0.7%	120 - 240
Levobupivacaine	0.5 – 0.75%	105 - 290
Ropivacaine	0.5 – 1%	90 -180

Table 1. Duration of sensory block for commonly used local anesthetics for epidural Anesthesia

4.1 Opioids

There is no single "best opioid" for epidural analgesia. Each opioid has a different set of pharmacologic properties that determine its effectiveness in a given clinical situation. One of the major properties of the opioids that affects their application for neuraxial analgesia is their lipid solubility (Figure 3). Lipophilic opioids such as sufentanil and fentanyl remain longer within the epidural space by partitioning into epidural fat and thus are found in lower concentrations in CSF than hydrophilic opioids such as morphine. Close titration of epidural local anesthetic and opioids concentrations must be performed to attain a balance between providing optimal analgesia and avoiding unwanted side effects.

5. Methods of drug delivery

Opioids or opioid-local anesthetic combinations can be administered in various methods. Patient-controlled epidural analgesia (PCEA) with a background infusion theoretically offers several advantages over continuous infusion or intermittent bolus methods. Background infusion provides fewer fluctuations in concentration of the analgesic drug, and the patient-controlled mode allows patients to control their analgesia on demand. Nevertheless, methods of drugs delivery also depend on an availability of equipment and the need for careful and repeated assessment by experienced staff. Common epidural regimens for PCEA or continuous infusion are listed in table 3.

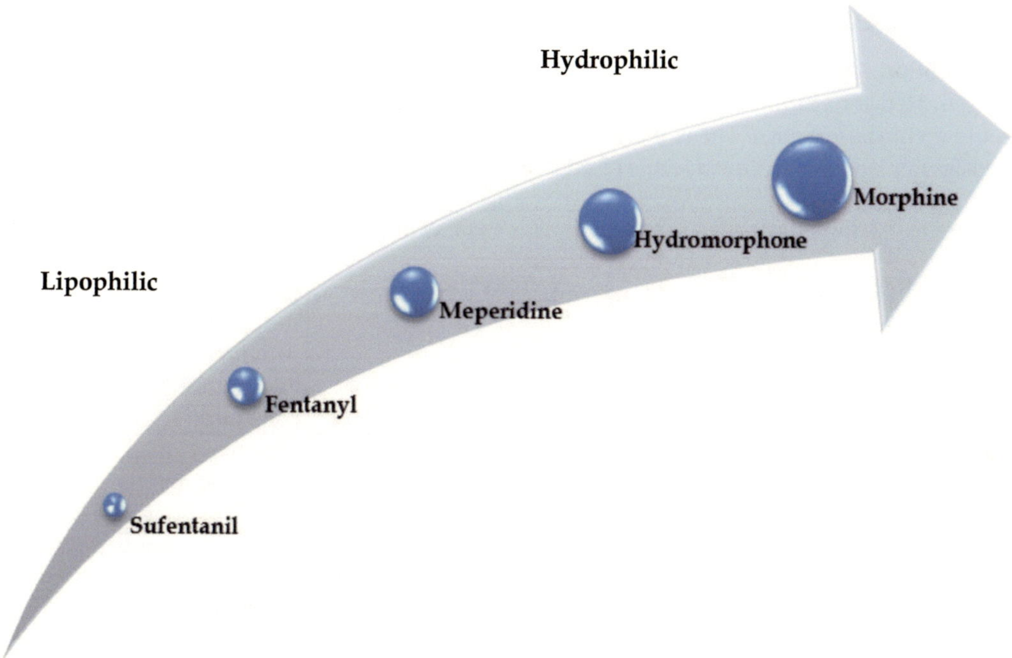

Fig. 3. The lipid solubility of the neuraxial opioids

Agent	Single bolus or intermittent injection		
	Dose	Onset (minutes)	Duration (hours)
Morphine	1-3 mg	20-60	8-24
Fentanyl	25-100 μg	4-10	4-6
Hydromorphone	0.1-0.3 mg	10-15	10-12

Table 2. Commonly used epidural opioids for single bolus or intermittent injection

Regimen	Continuous infusion	PCEA	
	Range (mL/ hour)	PCEA dose (mL.)	Lockout interval (minutes)
0.0625% bupivacaine + morphine 25-50 μg/mL	5-15 mL/h	1	10
0.0625% bupivacaine + fentanyl 1-10 μg/mL	5-15 mL/h	1	20
0.0625% bupivacaine + hydromorphone 3-12 μg/mL	5-15 mL/h	1	20

Table 3. Common epidural regimens

6. Adjuvant drugs

In addition to local anesthetics and opioids, other categories of agents have been investigated for epidural analgesia. All of the following drugs are not part of treatment in routine clinical practice. These include ketamine, clonidine, dexmedetomidine, midazolam, neosigmine and adrenaline. Details of adjuvant drugs are presented in table 4.

Reference	Adjuvant drugs	Dose or concentration	Type of surgery	Results
9	Ketamine	0.4 mg/ mL	Major surgery	Adding Ketamine to routine PCEA regimen provided lower pain score and reduced analgesic consumption.
10	Clonidine	20 µg/ hr	Gynecologic surgery	Improved analgesia during coughing, but was associated with hypotension and bradycardia.
11	Adrenaline	2 µg/ mL	Major surgery	Decrease pain while coughing.
12	Dexmedetomidine (single dose)	1.5 µg/ kg	Vaginal hysterectomy	Provide early onset of sensory analgesia, adequate sedation and prolonged postoperative analgesia when compared to clonidine.
13	Neostigmine	4 µg/ mL	Painless labor	Reduced the hourly bupivacaine requirement.
14	Midazolam (intermittent)	3 mg every 2 hours	Gastrectomy or cholecystectomy	Provide better analgesia, amnesia and sedation than bupivacaine alone.

Table 4. Types and results of adjuvant drugs on epidural analgesia

7. Complications associated with thoracic epidural analgesia

Most complications of TEA are not limited to the thoracic approach. Undesirable effects can occur during either the intraoperative or postoperative periods. In this chapter, complications are categorized into medication-related complications and risks of the thoracic epidural approach.

7.1 Medication-related complications

7.1.1 Complications associated with epidural opioids

Postoperative nausea and vomiting (PONV)

PONV is common, ranging from 3 to 60%. The first factor affecting this unpleasant effect of opioids is the type of opioid as the use of fentanyl is associated with a lower incidence of

PONV than the use of morphine. Secondly, PONV appears to be dose dependent, with lower doses related to lower incidences. Others risk factors of PONV are the female gender, a nonsmoker and a history of PONV. If patients have a high risk of PONV, 4 mg of dexamethasone and an additional antiemetic (12.5 to 25 mg of promethazine, 31.25 to 62.5 mg of dimenhydrinate, or 25 to 50 mg of metoclopramide) are recommended.

Pruritus

The incidence of pruritus ranges from 2 to 38%. Agents that have been used for the prevention and treatment of neuraxial opioid-induced pruritus are opioid antagonists, droperidol, propofol and serotonin receptor antagonists. (Richman & Wu, 2007)

Respiratory effects

Two types of desaturation usually occur after upper abdominal surgery. Constant desaturation has been attributed mainly to a decrease in functional residual capacity by atelectasis, reduction of the diaphragm and intercostal muscle activity, residual anesthetic drugs, and postoperative pain. Episodic desaturation may be related to a disruption of the normal sleep pattern induced by stress from the surgery and anesthesia. Both conditions frequently occur on the second postoperative day and may last longer than a week. A prospective study designed to determine the incidence of desaturation after upper abdominal surgery during the first 48 hours showed that desaturation occurred in 65 out of 171 patients (38%), and risk factors were obesity, epidural analgesia and subcostal incision. Based on the findings, it is reasonable that supplemental oxygen be given to patients undergoing upper abdominal surgery and that neuraxial opioids be administered for at least 48 hours postoperatively. (Siriussawakul et al., 2010)

7.2 Complications associated with local anesthetics

Hypotension

Hypotension from TEA is due to the local anesthetic induced sympathetic blockade, which causes a decrease in systemic vascular resistance and also attenuates the normal cardiac compensatory mechanism. Other causes of hypotension, such as low intravascular volume, bleeding and low cardiac output, must be considered when hypotension occurs. Volume loading (≥ 500 ml.) is frequently utilized prior to performing TEA. Atropine and vasopressor should be used to keep the patient's blood pressure at baseline.

Motor block

The use of local anesthetics for epidural analgesia may result in a lower extremity motor block, and this may lead to the development of pressure sores in the heel. A lower concentration of local anesthetics and TEA may decrease the incidence of motor block. A persistent or increasing motor block should be evaluated promptly if the motor block does not resolve after stopping the epidural infusion for approximately 2 hours.

Local anesthetic systemic toxicity

Local anesthetic systemic toxicity (LAST) results from an unintentional intravascular injection or the rapid absorption of the drugs into the circulation. The target of toxicity is the central nervous system (CNS) and the cardiovascular system (CVS). The CNS is more sensitive to LAST than the CVS. The clinical feature of intoxication has two stages: excitation and inhibition. CNS toxicity symptoms begin with a numbness of the tongue or circumoral structures, light-headedness, tinnitus, slurring of the speech, muscle twitching or tonic-clonic seizure, followed by drowsiness, a loss of consciousness and apnea. CVS intoxication symptoms are brief tachycardia and hypertension, followed by bradycardia and cardiovascular collapse. The recommendations to minimize the risk of LAST are using a test dose, administering the lowest drug concentration, and close monitoring for signs and symptoms during slow drug injection.

Urinary retention

Urinary retention may be associated with both local anesthetics and opioids interfering with detrusor muscle contraction and decreasing the sensation of urgency. Bladder function impairment will resolve when the block has regressed to the third sacral segment. Use of TEA, a low infusion rate and a low concentration of continuous epidural analgesia may result in a low incidence of urinary retention and diminish the need for bladder catheterization.

7.3 Risks of thoracic epidural approaches

Close proximity of the spinal cord, a narrower epidural space and a thinner ligamentum flavum make TEA more intimidating than via lumbar epidural approaches. Nevertheless, the placement of thoracic epidural catheters is relatively safe. There is no evidence of a higher incidence of neurologic complication compared to the placement of lumbar epidural catheters. Giebler et al report complications related to thoracic epidural catheterization in 4,185 patients. The overall incidence in this study was 3.1%. Adverse events included unsuccessful catheter placement, inadvertent dural puncture, postoperative radicular pain and peripheral nerve lesions (peroneal nerve palsy probably related to surgical position). There was no report of epidural hematoma or permanent sensory or motor defects. (Giebler et al, 1997) There were a few reports of an accidental intrapleural catheter placement and pneumothorax. (Cordone et al., 2007)

8. Conclusion

Epidural analgesia provides favorable outcomes after upper abdominal surgery. The success and safety of the procedure rely on expertise in the procedural, pharmacologic and physiologic aspects of epidural technique.

9. Appendix: Postoperative order for TEA

Thoracic Epidural Analgesia Order (Adult)
Name: .... Date: .... Diagnosis: .... Age: .... Weight: ....
Site of catheter insertion:

Access: ❑ Median ❑Paramedian

Injection level: T...

Catheter length in space: ....cm. Mark at skin: ....cm

Method of drug delivery:

❑ Single shot

Opioid: ❑ Morphine ❑ Fentanyl ❑ Other ....

Local anesthetic: ❑ Bupivacaine ❑ Levobupivacaine ❑ Ropivacaine ❑ Other ....

Concentration ....% Loading dose .... ml Loading time ....

❑ Intermittent

	First dose	Second dose	Third dose	Forth dose
Time				
Opioids - Type - Dose				
Local anesthetics - Concentration (%) - Loading dose (mL)				
Signature				

❑ Continuous epidural

❑ Local anesthetic: ....% ....mL

❑ Addition: ❑ Morphine...... mg./ mL ❑ Fentanyl ....µg/ mL ❑ Other.............

Infusion rate: .... mL/ hr

❑ Patient control epidural analgesia (PCEA)

Opioid : ❑ Morphine ❑ Fentanyl ❑ Other...

Local anesthetic:❑ Bupivacaine ❑ Levobupivacaine ❑ Ropivacaine ❑ Other...........

Concentration .... Loading dose .... mL.

Loading time ....Basal rate ....mL/ hr PCEA rate ....mL/ hr

Lockout interval...........................minutes 4 hour limit...............mL

Orders for monitoring and management of adverse effects
Respiratory monitoring - Record respiratory rate every hour for the first 12 h, every 2 h for the next 12 h, then every 4 hours until discontinue treatment. - Notify acute pain service immediately, for respiratory rate less than 6/ minute, place supplemental oxygen 8- 10 LPM via oxygen mask with bag and administer naloxone 0.2 mg IV repeat dose every 5 minute if respiratory rate less than 6/ minute
Inadequate analgesia (Numerical rating scale ≥ 4) ❑ Pethidine 20 mg IV prn q 2h ❑ Other .... ❑ Notify acute pain service
Nausea and vomiting ❑ Ondansetron ❑4 mg ❑8 mg IV prn q 8h ❑ Metoclopramide .... mg IV prn q 6h ❑ Other ....
Pruritus ❑ Diphenhydramine (25 mg/ 10 ml or cap) ❑ Syrup 10 mL ❑ 1 cap oral prn q 6h ❑ Chlorpheniramine 10 mg IV prn q 6h ❑ Other ....
Urinary retention ❑ Keep indwelling urinary catheter in place until discontinuation of epidural analgesia ❑ Other..

10. References

van Lier F, van der Geest PJ, Hoeks SE, van Gestel YR, Hol JW, Sin DD, Stolker RJ, Poldermans D. (2011) Epidural analgesia is associated with improved health outcomes of surgical patients with chronic obstructive pulmonary disease. *Anesthesiology.* Vol.115 (2):pp.315-21.

Hurley RW and Wu CL.(2009).Acute Postoperative Pain. In:. *Miller's Anesthesia, 7th ed.* Ronald D. Miller.pp.2757-2781. Churchill Livingstone, Philadelphia:

Neal JM. (2004). Epidural Anesthesia. In: *Regional anesthesia: the requisites in anesthesiology*.Rathmell JP, Neal JM and Viscomi CM. pp.99-113.: Mosby, Inc., Philadephia

Gray AT. (2010).*Atlas of ultrasound-guided regional anesthesia*. Elsevier Inc, Philadephia.

Moore D, Batra M. (1981) The components of and effective test dose prior to epidural block. *Anesthesiology*. Vol55 : pp.693.

Minzter BH, Johnson RF, Grimm BJ. (2002). The practice of thoracic epidural analgesia: a survey of academic medical centers in the United States. *Anesth Analg*. Vol.95: pp. 472-5

Conacher ID, Slinger PD. (2003) Pain Management. In: *Thoracic Anesthesia, 3rdedition*.Kaplan JA, Slinger PD. pp.436-462. Churchill Livingstone, Philadelphia.

Cok OY, Eker HE, Turkoz A, Findikcioglu A, Akin S, Aribogan A, Arslan G. (2001)Thoracic epidural anesthesia and analgesia during the perioperative period of thoracic surgery : levobupivacaine versus bupivacaine. *J Cardiothrac Vasc Anesth* . Vol.25:pp.449-54.

Chia YY, Liu K, Liu YC, Chang HC, Wong CS. (1998). Adding ketamine in a multimodal patient-controlled epidural regimen reduces postoperative pain and analgesic consumption. *Anesth Analg*. Vol.86(6):pp.1245-9.

Paech MJ, Pavy TJ, Orlikowski CE, Lim W, Evans SF.(1997). Postoperative epidural infusion: a randomized, double-blind, dose-finding trial of clonidine in combination with bupivacaine and fentanyl. *Anesth Analg*. Vol 84 (6) : pp.1323-8.

Niemi G, Breivik H. (2003). The minimally effective concentration of adrenaline in a low-concentration thoracic epidural analgesic infusion of bupivacaine, fentanyl and adrenaline after major surgery. A randomized, double-blind, dose-finding study. *Acta Anaesthesiol Scand*. Vol.47(4):pp.439-50.

Bajwa SJ, Bajwa SK, Kaur J, Singh G, Arora V, Gupta S, Kulshrestha A, Singh A, Parmar S, Singh A, Goraya S.(2011). Dexmedetomidine and clonidine in epidural anaesthesia: A comparative evaluation. *Indian J Anaesth*. Vol.55(2):pp116-21.

Ross VH, Pan PH, Owen MD, Seid MH, Harris L, Clyne B, Voltaire M, Eisenach JC. (2009).Neostigmine decreases bupivacaine use by patient-controlled epidural analgesia during labor: a randomized controlled study. *Anesth Analg*. Vol.109(2):pp524-31.

Nishiyama T, Matsukawa T, Hanaoka K. (1999) Continuous epidural administration of midazolam and bupivacaine for postoperative analgesia. *Acta Anaesthesiol Scand*. Vol. 43(5):pp.568-72.

Richman JM and Wu CL. (2007).Complications associated with continuous epidural analgesia. In: *Complication in regional anesthesia & pain medicine*. Neal JM and Rathmell JP. pp. 177-193.Elsevier Inc, Philadelphia.

Siriussawakul A, Mandee S, Thonsontia J, Vitayaburananont P, Areewatana S, Laonarinthawoot J.(2010) Obesity, epidural analgesia, and subcostal incision are risk factors for postoperative desaturation. *Can J Anaest*. Vol; 57(5):pp.415-22.

Giebler RM, Scherer RU, Peter J.(1997). Incidence of neurologic complications related to thoracic epidural catheterization. *Anesthesiology*. Vol. 86(1): pp.55-63.

Cordone MA, Wu CL, Maceda AL, Richman JM. (2007). Unrecognized contralateral intrapleural catheter: bilateral blockade may obscure detection of failed epidural catheterization. *Anesth Analg*. Vol.104(3):pp.735-7.

5

The Impact of Epidural Analgesia on Postoperative Outcome After Major Abdominal Surgery

Iulia Cindea, Alina Balcan, Viorel Gherghina, Bianca Samoila, Dan Costea, Catalin Grasa and Gheorghe Nicolae
Emergency Clinical Hospital of Constantza, Romania

1. Introduction

Despite the spread of minimally invasive surgical techniques and improvements in postoperative management, major abdominal procedures still induce neurohumoral changes responsible for postoperative pain, various organ dysfunctions, prolonged hospitalization and convalescence.

One of the main concerns of patients presenting for major abdominal surgery and anesthesiologists involved in postoperative care is postoperative analgesia. The most common postoperative pain control methods are epidural infusion of a combination of local anesthetic and an opioid or local anesthetic alone and administration of intravenous opiates, both of them being accepted options following major abdominal procedures.

Parenteral opioids can provide adequate analgesia but pain on movement is generally less controlled. Their side-effects, in particular respiratory depression, limit the dose that can be given, therefore resulting in suboptimal analgesia for some subjects.

Epidural analgesia confers excellent pain relief and complete dynamic analgesia leading to a substantial reduction in the surgical stress response. Epidural analgesia seems to provide favorable effects on coagulation and homeostasis, as well as on cardio-respiratory, gastrointestinal and immune functions, all these potential positive influences being theoretically translated into an improved quality of patient recovery.

The outcome of different treatment methods for postoperative pain after major abdominal surgery has been an issue of controversy, mainly because of the increasingly need for large patient numbers in any individual trial in order to derive reliable conclusions. Epidural analgesia is the most investigated strategy, being assumed that it has the greatest theoretical potential to considerably modify postoperative outcome.

This chapter systematically reviews a large-scale data to acquire suitable evidence on the effects of epidural analgesia on postoperative outcome, contributing to the collaborative efforts of anesthesiologists and surgeons for the improvement of patient recovery after major abdominal surgery.

2. Method for systematic review

A broad search strategy including Medline and Cochrane Library databases has been conducted. Meta-analyses and large controlled trials that randomized major abdominal surgery patients to either epidural or opioid-based systemic analgesia and that are reported on postoperative outcomes have been retrieved. All references within relevant papers have been further checked for additional studies.

The above mentioned data sources have been searched from January 1990 to December 2010, our investigation being limited to the last two decades because of progress of surgical techniques, improvement in quality of postoperative care and implementation of rational use of aggressive pain control.

The following search terms have been used in various combinations: major abdominal surgery, postoperative pain, postoperative analgesia, epidural analgesia, patient-controlled analgesia, postoperative complications, pulmonary complications, respiratory insufficiency, pneumonia, myocardial ischemia, myocardial infarction, heart failure, dysrhythmias, ileus, infection, surgical wound infection, deep venous thrombosis, cognitive disorders, postoperative mortality, cost-efficiency ratio, postoperative stress response, risks of epidural analgesia, duration of hospital stay.

Firstly, the trials have been screened per inclusion and exclusion criteria. Secondly, all the inclusion criteria have been validated for the accepted studies before the data extraction process. In those cases in which uncertainty arose, the articles to be excluded have been validated, too.

According to the study design, the selected trials have been stratified into levels of evidence ranged from I to IV where level I: systematic review of randomized controlled trials, level II: randomized controlled trials, level III: non-randomized controlled trials or from cohort or case-control analytical studies and level IV: expert opinion.

Trials in adult patients in which epidural analgesia has been started immediately postoperatively and has been maintained for 3 days after surgery, have been included. The included studies have tested thoracic or lumbar epidurals, the analgesic regimen consisting of local anesthetic alone or a combination of local anesthetic and opioids. Controls have received subcutaneous, intravenous or intramuscular opioids that have been given on demand, regularly or via patient-controlled analgesia.

Considering that best evidence is coming from large patient numbers, preference has been given to the large sample sizes. Consequently, we have chosen an $n \geq 100$ (100 individuals per randomized group) as suitable inclusion criterion for individual studies. This option is based on highest reported incidences of postoperative morbidity to maximize capture of randomized controlled trials.

We have noted the type of epidural analgesia involving the level of catheter insertion, duration and analgesic regimen. For systemic analgesia, the route of administration and the regimen have been recorded, too. Definitions of postoperative outcome parameters have been taken as reported in the original articles.

Those trials in which controls have received epidural analgesia or have not received systemic opioids have been rejected. Trials with fewer than 100 patients per group have been excluded, too. Studies which data on postoperative outcome assessment could not be extracted have been considered out of the interest of this analysis.

Based on these criteria we have selected the eligible meta-analyses, systematic reviews, randomized controlled trials and observational database articles to gather evidence on the impact of epidural analgesia on postoperative outcome in major abdominal surgery patients.

3. Effects of epidural analgesia on major postoperative outcomes

3.1 Effect of epidural analgesia on pulmonary function

Postoperative pulmonary dysfunction after major abdominal surgery has a multifactorial pathophysiology including deranged central ventilatory control, alteration of normal respiratory muscle activity, diaphragmatic dysfunction, consequence of a reflex inhibition of phrenic nerve activity and postoperative pain that contributes to the impairment of pulmonary mechanics (Liu & Wu, 2007; Nimmo, 2004). From far, the most important effect of major abdominal surgery on pulmonary function is the reduction of functional residual capacity (FRC) determined by diaphragmatic dysfunction, pain-related reduction of spontaneous ventilation and decreased chest wall compliance (Moraca et al., 2003; Warner, 2000).

Postoperative pulmonary complications, as common as cardiac complications in the context of major abdominal surgery, may prolong the duration of hospitalization and carry an increased risk of mortality. Epidural analgesia confers optimal postoperative pain control thus resulting in pain-free ventilation, coughing and better cooperation with physiotherapy (Wu et al., 2005).

On the other hand, the superior pain relief provided by this technique reduces the consumption of parenteral opioids that adversely affect ventilation and gas exchange (Nimmo, 2004).

The interruption of the reflex inhibition of phrenic nerve by segmental block is likely to have a beneficial effect, mainly by allowing normal diaphragm function, thus improving diaphragmatic activity (Liu & Wu, 2007; Nimmo, 2004).

Epidural analgesia obtunds the stress response to major surgery, fact that is of particular interest for the clinician, since it reduces the level of postoperative immunosuppression, thus contributing to decrease of pulmonary infections incidence (Nimmo, 2004).

Taking into account that the effects on respiratory muscle function are complex, it has been suggested that epidural analgesia for pulmonary function might be unfavorable during early postoperative period due to potential paralysis of intercostals or abdominals and changes in bronchial tone (Liu & Wu, 2007; Waurick & Van Aken, 2005). However, it has been demonstrated that epidural analgesia does not impair respiratory muscle strength or airway flow even in patients with end-stage chronic obstructive pulmonary disease, resulting, by contrast, in better ventilatory mechanics and optimal respiratory muscle force generation (Groeben et al., 2002; Gruber et al., 2001; Waurick & Van Aken, 2005).

Even the biological basis underlying these associations is unclear, it is well documented that epidural analgesia improves some measurable pulmonary function parameters such as tidal volume, vital capacity, forced vital capacity at 24 hours, forced expiratory volume in 1 second at 24 hours, peak expiratory flow rate at 24 hours. It has been noted a significantly increased arterial oxygen pressure at 24 and 72 hours, too (Moraca et al., 2003; Pöpping et al., 2008).

However, it should be noted that, there is no documented significant correlation between postoperative pulmonary function tests and the incidence of pulmonary complications (Ballantyne et al., 1998; Kehlet & Holte, 2001; Moraca et al., 2003).

Therefore, such surrogate outcome measures seem to be inappropriate for the investigation of postoperative pulmonary morbidity. Other markers, namely the incidence of pneumonia respiratory failure, atelectasis and hypoxemia have been demonstrated to be more adequate in this respect (Kehlet & Holte, 2001; Moraca et al., 2003).

Thus, large meta-analyses of randomized controlled trials pointed out a significant reduction in pneumonia, as well as in respiratory depression in major abdominal surgery subjects treated postoperatively with epidural analgesia, compared with those receiving systemic analgesia (PCA) (Liu & Wu, 2007; Moraca et al., 2003). This finding is in agreement with other studies that noted a significantly decreased risk of respiratory failure associated with epidural analgesia for patients undergoing major abdominal procedures (Jiang et al., 2005; Park et al., 2001; Rigg et al., 2002; Werawatganon & Charuluxananan, 2005).

An earlier meta-analysis on randomized clinical trials examining the use of epidural analgesia in major abdominal surgery concluded that this technique significantly reduces the incidence of pulmonary complications overall, being specifically associated with significantly less atelectasis and pneumonia (Ballantyne et al., 1998; Moraca et al., 2003).

Over the last decade, the protective effect of epidural analgesia on postoperative pulmonary complications has decreased, compared with conventional systemic analgesia. This phenomenon does not seem to be related to a decrease in the efficacy of the epidurals per se, but rather to a reduction in baseline risk of such complications. Modification of standard care in patients undergoing major abdominal procedures including respiratory physiotherapy, the routine use of naso-gastric tube, prophylactic antibiotics and early mobilization, may all have favorably influenced the risk of pulmonary complications (Pöpping et al., 2008).

In conclusion, consistent data from meta-analyses and large randomized controlled trials support the potential physiologic benefit of epidural analgesia for reducing postoperative pulmonary complications in major abdominal surgery patients.

3.2 Effect of epidural analgesia on postoperative pain

Adequate postoperative pain control is a key therapeutic component of the complex multimodal rehabilitation program after major abdominal procedures (Bartha et al., 2006). In this context, epidural technique is considered by many the standard-care strategy, because it provides complete analgesia and especially effective dynamic pain relief. Such postoperative benefits allow the subject to early mobilize and resume normal activities (Block et al., 2003; Dolin et al., 2002). The optimal level of postoperative analgesia is usually achieved with a combination of epidural local anesthetic and opioid (Kehlet, 1994, 1997; Nimmo, 2004; Wheatley et al., 2001).

The comparison of epidural therapy versus systemic opioids after major abdominal surgery, that has been studied in many individual trials and has been reviewed in large meta-analyses, has pointed out that the epidural technique provided a significantly better analgesia at all time points up to the third postoperative day (Waurick & Van Aken, 2005).

Large-scale observational data acquired from systematic reviews comprising large number of patients have noted that postoperative epidural analgesia was associated with significantly lower incidence of severe and moderate pain by comparison to systemic opioids strategy, after major abdominal procedures (Waurick & Van Aken, 2005).

"Preemptive analgesia" is an attractive concept revealing that blockade of nociception by epidural analgesia before surgical manipulation will positively affect the perception of subsequent painful stimuli. Thus, pain perception and overall analgesic needs could significantly decrease during hospitalization and the incidence of long-term pain after major abdominal procedures might be reduced in patients treated with preemptive epidural analgesia. Despite encouraging findings from small clinical trials, this effect has not been reproduced in other studies. The validity and clinical relevance of preemptive epidural analgesia is still controversial and more trials investigating the effect of this technique on either acute or chronic pain after major abdominal surgery are warranted (Kehlet & Dahl, 2003; Moraca et al., 2003).

Clearly, epidural strategy is associated with a statistically significant and clinically relevant improvement of postoperative pain control in patients undergoing major abdominal surgery, although it requires specific technical and pharmacological skills, as well as professional monitoring of the subjects.

3.3 Effect of epidural analgesia on gastrointestinal function

Gastrointestinal paralysis, nausea and vomiting recognized as common clinical problems after major abdominal surgery may last for days and prolong hospitalization and convalescence. Although the pathophysiology of postoperative ileus is multifactorial, primary mechanisms include local inflammatory response, nociceptive reflexes, activation of inhibitory splanchnic reflexes and systemically applied opioids, all of these being subject to modification by postoperative epidural analgesia (Kehlet & Holte, 2001; Liu & Wu, 2007; Nimmo, 2004; Waurick & Van Aken, 2005).

After major abdominal procedures, epidural analgesia provides superior pain control by blocking nociceptive reflexes, thus limiting systemic opioids use, a documented factor that increases the risk of ileus (Liu & Wu, 2007; Wu et al., 2005). The sympathetic block from epidural analgesia may attenuate postoperative reflex inhibition of gastrointestinal motility thus reducing the duration of ileus and allowing early enteral feeding (Bauer & Boeckxstaens, 2004; Jørgensen et al., 2000; Mythen, 2005). Attenuation of the stress response to major abdominal surgery reduces the inflammatory response that contributes to the maintenance of postoperative ileus (Mythen, 2005; Nimmo, 2004).

There has been debate about whether the ileus-reducing effect associated with postoperative epidural analgesia may pose a risk to the integrity of intestinal anastomoses. Data from published randomized clinical studies and large meta-analyses have consistently indicated that thoracic epidural analgesia, suitable after major abdominal surgery, blocks the activity of sympathetic fibres innervating the mesenterial blood vessels, thus improving the mucosal blood flow, even under circumstances of reduced perfusion pressure. In this way, postoperative epidural analgesia could contribute to healing rather than to anastomotic dehiscence when compared to systemic opioid analgesia (Kehlet & Holte, 2001; Liu & Wu, 2007; Waurick & Van Aken, 2005).

In summary postoperative epidural analgesia significantly reduces postoperative ileus, with major clinical impact allowing early recovery of gut function, subsequently early enteral nutrition with beneficial effect on postoperative nitrogen balance and total body protein preservation, thus resulting in better outcome.

The great majority of randomized clinical trials investigated have demonstrated a significant reduction in postoperative ileus with epidural technique by comparison to systemic opioid analgesia (Kehlet & Holte, 2001; Waurick & Van Aken, 2005).

3.4 Effect of epidural analgesia on stress response to major abdominal surgery

The postoperative stress response to major abdominal surgery is defined as a cascade of effects that result from activation of neural, metabolic and endocrine pathways with initiation of coagulation and inflammatory mechanisms (Nimmo, 2004).

This postoperative surgical stress response could contribute to various organ dysfunctions in susceptible individuals, thus leading to a difficult and prolonged recovery and rehabilitation (Kehlet & Holte, 2001). There is a common consensus that a reduction in the stress response is followed by a reduced postoperative major morbidity and improved surgical outcome (Holte & Kehlet, 2002; Kehlet & Holte, 2001; Nimmo, 2004).

It has been postulated that pain relief represents an effective method to reduce surgical stress response, since afferent neural stimuli and activation of autonomic nervous system together with other reflexes by pain serve as a major release mechanism of the endocrine and metabolic responses (Kehlet & Holte, 2001). Thus, one of the beneficial effects of epidural analgesia results from obtunding the postoperative stress response by provision of optimal analgesia.

However, the efficacy in modulating endocrine-metabolic response substantially depends on the level of epidural blockade, its duration, the analgesic regimen (local anesthetic-based regimen or local anesthetic-opioid combination regimen), as well as the administration technique (continuous epidural analgesia or patient-controlled postoperative epidural analgesia) and the literature has been confounded by high heterogeneity in this respect. Thus, many reported randomized studies with different analgesia regimens have been combined in meta-analyses, furthermore often there is no distinction between thoracic and lumbar epidural blockade or various techniques of administration, facts that limit the interpretation of these findings (Grass, 2000; Kehlet & Holte, 2001; Wheatley et al., 2001).

However, use of epidural analgesia to reduce the deleterious effects of postoperative stress response has been demonstrated to improve the clinical outcome, becoming a popular strategy in major abdominal surgery patients.

3.5 Effect of epidural analgesia on muscle function

Epidural analgesia is particularly effective at providing complete pain relief at movement (Nimmo, 2004; Wheatley et al., 2001). On the other hand, alteration of postoperative stress response has been shown to reduce postoperative catabolism resulting in less muscle wasting and postoperative weakness (Nimmo, 2004; Rigg et al., 2002; Wheatley et al., 2001).

These effects in conjunction with early postoperative feeding could contribute to muscle strength and an improved exercise tolerance, allowing the patient to sit out of bed, even on the day of surgery and to actively mobilize next day (Holte & Kehlet, 2002; Nimmo, 2004).

Conclusively, there is general agreement that epidural analgesia has positive effect on postoperative mobilization, faster physical rehabilitation being recognized as a prerequisite for early postoperative recovery after major abdominal surgery.

3.6 Effect of epidural analgesia on cardiovascular function

Postoperative cardiovascular complications, a major cause of postoperative death, are typically reported after major abdominal procedures, particularly in elderly that carry a high risk for such events (Liu & Wu, 2007).

Poorly controlled postoperative pain and stress response lead to sympathetic arousal that increases myocardial oxygen demand by increasing heart rate, arterial blood pressure and contractility (Nygärd et al., 2005). In addition, sympathetic activation could decrease myocardial oxygen supply by enhancing the risk of thromboembolic complications, especially coronary thrombosis (Devereaux et al., 2005; Waurick & Van Aken, 2005).

Thoracic epidural analgesia reduces sympathetic activity, providing a favorable balance of myocardial oxygen. Thus, thoracic epidural analgesia improves myocardial blood flow by selectively increasing the diameter of stenotic epicardial coronary arteries while maintaining coronary perfusion pressure, and decreases myocardial oxygen demand by reducing pain, heart rate and systemic vascular resistance (Liu & Wu, 2007; Peyton et al., 2003; Waurick & Van Aken, 2005).

Procedure-specific meta-analyses and randomized controlled trials have been focused on the role of postoperative epidural analgesia compared to standard intravenous treatment in terms of cardiac protection after major abdominal procedures. Thus, subjects with thoracic epidural analgesia have experienced lower number of ischemic episodes of shorter duration, a significant reduction in the incidence of myocardial infarction, heart failure and dysrhythmias (Beattie et al., 2001; Block et al., 2003; Kehlet & Holte, 2001; Waurick & Van Aken, 2005).

Reaching valid conclusions based on these findings could be difficult because of differences in definitions of cardiovascular adverse events, the use of different analgesic techniques and regimens and the inadequately sized studies to analyze cardiovascular complications (Kehlet & Holte, 2001; Liu & Wu, 2007).

Regardless the above-mentioned limits, we have found enough evidence to suggest a clinically relevant benefit of epidural analgesia and thoracic epidural analgesia in particular, in reduction of postoperative cardiac morbidity after major abdominal surgery, the largest improvement being observed in cardiac high-risk patients (Liu & Wu, 2007; Waurick & Van Aken, 2005).

In summary, although the impact on cardiac morbidity continues to demand our attention, the clinically significant advantages of postoperative epidural block after major abdominal procedures have been demonstrated particularly in specific categories of subjects bearing preoperative cardiovascular co-morbidities.

3.7 Effect of epidural analgesia on coagulation

The coagulation-fibrinolysis balance is disturbed in association with major abdominal procedures (Liu & Wu, 2007). Thus, after surgical incision there have been identified high plasma levels of tissue factor, tissue plasminogen activator, plasminogen activator inhibitor-1, von Willebrand factor which lead to a hypercoagulability and hypofibrinolytic state with resultant risk of formation of deep venous thrombosis and potentially fatal pulmonary embolism (Agnelli, 2004; Bombeli & Spahn, 2004; Liu & Wu, 2007; Roderick et al., 2005). Use of effective methods of thromboprophylaxis in surgical practice makes difficult the estimation of current incidences of deep venous thrombosis and pulmonary embolism (Liu & Wu, 2007).

Epidural analgesia provides potential benefits such as reduction of coagulation proteins and platelet activity, preservation of fibrinolytic function by obtunding the postoperative stress response and increase of arterial and venous blood flow, thus preventing postoperative coagulation-related complications (Kehlet & Holte, 2001; Liu & Wu, 2007; Moraca et al., 2003). Early postoperative mobilization facilitated by dynamic analgesia could play a protective role, too (Nimmo, 2004).

However, systematic reviews of randomized clinical trials in major abdominal surgery have indicated a non-significant reduction of thromboembolic complications, assessed by phlebography or iodine-fibrinogen scans, when postoperative epidural analgesic regimen is compared with systemic opioid technique (Kehlet & Holte, 2001; Liu & Wu, 2007).

Furthermore, another specific analysis of randomized studies has been noted, beside the extremely low incidences of thromboembolic complications due to thromboprophylaxis, no differences between groups with epidural analgesia and those with systemic opioids, after major abdominal procedures (Kehlet & Holte, 2001; Liu & Wu, 2007).

In conclusion, in the era of rapidly evolving strategies of effective thromboprophylaxis in the field of major abdominal surgery, there is minimal evidence that epidural analgesia could attenuate the risk of postoperative coagulation-related complications.

3.8 Effect of epidural analgesia on immune function

Major abdominal surgery is associated with an imbalance between proinflammatory and antiinflammatory cytokines and immunocompetent cells in favor of an early hyperinflammatory response (Sido et al., 2004). The immune system impairment determined by extensive tissue damage, anesthesia and uncontrolled postoperative pain, consist of release of tumor necrosis factor α, interleukin-1, interleukin-2, interleukin-6, neutrophil activation, polymorphonuclear and macrophage oxidative activity, lead to a significant cell-mediated immunosuppression manifested by monocyte deactivation and phagocytes inhibition (Liu & Wu, 2007; Yokoyama et al., 2005).

Epidural analgesia could improve postoperative immune function, at least theoretically, by reducing proinflammatory response as well as lymphocyte suppression (Beilin et al., 2003; Liu & Wu, 2007; Waurick & Van Aken, 2005). The studies that have investigated the effect of epidural analgesia compared to systemic opioid regimen on postoperative immune function in major abdominal surgery patients, have noted reduced suppression of lymphocyte proliferation and attenuated proinflammatory response (Beilin et al., 2003; Yokoyama et al., 2005).

Insufficient controlled postoperative pain may increase adrenergic nerve activity and plasma catecholamine concentration leading to peripheral vasoconstriction, reduced perfusion and decreased tissue oxygen partial pressure. As a consequence, peripheral tissues suffer of hypoxia that is associated with an increased incidence of surgical wound infections (Kabon et al., 2003; Waurick & Van Aken, 2005).

Postoperative epidural analgesia substantially diminishes sympato-adrenergic response caused by nociceptive stimuli improving microcirculation and tissue oxygen partial pressure and thus might promote wound healing (Kabon et al., 2003).

Despite the improvement of postoperative immune function and tissue oxygen tension, the potential benefit of epidural analgesia on resistance to infectious complications, in particular to surgical wound infections is clinically irrelevant (Liu & Wu, 2007).

In conclusion, there is clinical minimal evidence suggesting that epidural analgesia positively affects the risk of postoperative infections, especially wound infections in major abdominal surgery patients, as few studies have specifically addressed this question.

3.9 Effect of epidural analgesia on cognitive function

Given the common occurrence and its long-term effects in functioning, especially in elderly, postoperative cognitive decline is a clinically important issue in postoperative management of major abdominal surgery patients (Fong et al., 2006; Liu & Wu, 2007; Moraca et al., 2003).

The etiology of cognitive dysfunction is still not elucidated and is probably multifactorial (Kehlet & Holte, 2001; Liu & Wu, 2007; Moraca et al., 2003). The cited studies do agree that preexisting patient factors, as well as intraoperative and postoperative causes are involved (Fong et al., 2006; Liu & Wu, 2007).

Taking into account that preoperative patient-related factors are not changeable and intraoperative anesthetic types have not been shown to affect mental status, there are reports that have been focused on postoperative management strategies, the rationale for this choice being the association between postoperative pain and cognitive decline (Fong et al., 2006; Moraca et al., 2003).

As epidural analgesia provides better pain relief and spares systemic opioids, there is at least a theoretical reason for improved cognitive status with this strategy after major abdominal surgery. However, the clinical impact of postoperative epidural analgesia on cognitive dysfunction after major abdominal procedures is controversial (Liu & Wu, 2007; Moraca et al., 2003).

There are studies that have not found any difference between epidural and parenteral analgesia with respect to postoperative cognitive decline. The small sample sizes and the lack of standardized approach for mental disorders monitoring could significantly limit the validity of such findings (Fong et al., 2006; Liu & Wu, 2007).

Conversely, in other studies epidural analgesia has been shown to cause better pain control with less sedation, thus contributing to a significant improvement in postoperative cognition when compared with intravenous opioids (Kehlet & Holte, 2001; Moraca et al., 2003).

Similar to the above-mentioned studies, these investigations are limited by small sample size, heterogeneous criteria to define postoperative cognitive dysfunction, variations in the level at which the epidural catheter is inserted, as well as the medication used, meaning local anesthetic or local anesthetic and opioid.

In conclusion, the effect of epidural analgesia on postoperative cognitive dysfunction is still unclear and the observations from this review reinforce the necessity for future investigations using appropriate and uniform outcome measures and, most importantly, enrolling a sufficient number of patients.

3.10 Effect of epidural analgesia on postoperative mortality

The increasing safety of current surgical procedures, together with advances in anesthetic and intensive-care practice lead to a substantial reduction in postoperative fatality, even in high-risk patients undergoing major abdominal surgery. Thus, the postoperative mortality as an end-point may not be adequate to demonstrate the benefits of epidural analgesia (Nimmo, 2004).

However, it has to be mentioned that a number of studies have investigated the effect of epidural analgesia versus standard systemic opioids on postoperative mortality in high-risk patients undergoing extensive abdominal surgery. Most of these trials have reported no significant reduction in postoperative mortality with epidural blockade (Kehlet & Holte, 2001; Liu & Wu, 2007; Nimmo, 2004). The criticized methodology and the small number of patients limit the interpretation of these findings.

It is of note an often-cited prospective randomized controlled study (MASTER study) that has found no difference in overall mortality between groups, but a reduced incidence of pulmonary and thromboembolic complications and significantly better analgesia in the epidural group (Liu & Wu, 2007; Nimmo, 2004; Rigg et al., 2000; Waurick & Van Aken, 2004). Once again this trial has been not adequately sized to assess mortality, a postoperative complication with currently low incidence and it proves insufficient evidence for valid conclusions in this respect (Liu & Wu, 2007).

Procedure-specific meta-analyses focused on the impact of epidural analgesia on postoperative mortality have shown a benefit, but because of the occurrence of fatal events in a few studies involving a minority of the total number of subjects, the validity and clinical relevance of these results is questioned (Liu & Wu, 2007; Nimmo, 2004).

Analysis of large-scale databases including patients undergoing a variety of extensive abdominal procedures has revealed the association of postoperative epidural analgesia with a significantly lower incidence for 7-day and 30-day mortality (Liu & Wu, 2007). Although the number of patients is impressive this time, such analyses suffer from the retrospective nature and degree of association between epidural analgesia and mortality as postoperative outcome (Liu & Wu, 2007).

In summary, our review of the literature suggests it is unlikely that any effect of epidural block translates into relevant improvement in postoperative mortality after major abdominal surgery.

3.11 Effect of epidural analgesia on duration of intensive care unit and hospital stay

Postoperative epidural analgesia after major abdominal procedures may induce improvements in many physiological variables, clinically translated into positive effects on paralytic ileus, pulmonary, cardiac and thromboembolic outcome. The reduction in the incidence and severity of postoperative morbidity suggests at least theoretically, a decrease in length of intensive care and hospital stay.

It is therefore surprising and somewhat disappointing that the effect of epidural analgesic techniques on duration of intensive care unit and hospital stay has been rather small or non-demonstrable by clinical trials.

Thus, large randomized studies prospectively enrolling high-risk patients undergoing major abdominal surgery have found no difference in length of stay in intensive care unit or in the hospital between subjects receiving postoperative epidural analgesia and those receiving iv opioids (Kehlet & Holte, 2001; Peyton et al., 2003).

Other studies have noted a discrepancy between earlier achievement of intensive care discharge criteria and actual hospital stay that is not affected in patients receiving epidural analgesia compared to those treated with systemic opioids after major abdominal surgery (Kehlet & Holte, 2001).

On the other hand, retrospective analyses have concluded that both intensive care unit and hospital length of stay have been decreased in patients treated with epidural analgesia compared to those treated with systemic opioids (Moraca et al., 2003; Rigg et al., 2002).

However, it should be emphasized that intensive care and hospital stay may be poor outcome measures since they depend on a lot of factors other than pain control and in order to demonstrate a potential reduction in their duration by epidural analgesia, this strategy has to be integrated into a multimodal rehabilitation program (Kehlet, 2008; Kehlet & Holte, 2001).

Although there is general agreement that epidural analgesia improves postoperative outcome in major abdominal surgery patients, the progress in reducing hospital and intensive care length of stay is slow (Kehlet, 2008; Kehlet & Wilmore, 2008).

Consequently, the well documented clinical advantages of epidural analgesia have to be used together with adjustments of postoperative care into a complex rehabilitation program to facilitate early recovery and the preliminary experience has shown a positive effect of such a collaborative efforts in reducing hospital and intensive care stay (Basse et al., 2000; Kehlet & Holte, 2001).

3.12 Effect of epidural analgesia on cost of postoperative care

An economic analysis on postoperative pain treatment comparing epidural analgesia and standard intravenous opioid analgesia after major abdominal surgery becomes of interest, especially when health-care resources are scarce. Apart from efficacy and safety, a policy decision in selecting different analgesia strategies should take into account cost-effectiveness ratio.

Although the costs per quality adjusted life year is recommended in the available health economic literature when performing cost-effectiveness evaluation, such a measure of outcome appears inadequate for our analysis, since this review is focused on a short effect duration of acute pain treatment. Thus, the cost per gained pain-free day has been considered appropriate under these circumstances, the cited studies being in complete agreement that postoperative pain control is a mandatory component of early postoperative care (Bartha et al., 2006).

On the other hand, for a rigorous economic evaluation there are many other relevant aspects of multidimensional experience of pain, that reflect the improved health state of subject due to pain relief. Thus, other outcome measures such as length of hospital stay, morbidity and mortality should be considered (McLeod et al., 2001; Paulsen et al., 2001; Werawatganon & Charuluxananan, 2005).

There are relatively few economic analyses of postoperative pain treatment after major abdominal procedures designed to estimate the cost-effectiveness of epidural analgesia compared with systemic opioids and the available studies have sample sizing and methodological limitations (Bartha et al., 2006). Beside all these difficulties, there is generally accepted that the cost of epidural analgesia is around three times higher than that of standard intravenous analgesia (Bartha et al., 2006). Here is a judgment of value whether this supplementary cost per pain-free day is reasonable in relation to the benefit.

Another problem to be taken into account before decision making is who will suffer because of lack of health-care (Bartha et al., 2006). Under actual circumstances of poor financial support, epidural analgesia as better choice for postoperative pain relief sometimes is not the best one. Thus, it seems reasonable to go to the second best alternative, systemic analgesia, that appears the most cost-effective analgesic modality (Bartha et al., 2006).

Before any conclusion concerning policy recommendations, such a difference in costs has to be judged closely related to parameters that have been largely ignored in previous research on health-care expenses, namely postoperative morbidity, mortality and duration of hospital stay after major abdominal surgery. This approach will help the clinical practitioner to answer the question whether epidural analgesia results in objective improvement in outcomes in major abdominal surgery patients and its related extra costs are outweighed by clinical benefits.

4. Complications of epidural analgesia

Epidural analgesia can be provided safely in patients undergoing major abdominal surgery since the documented risk-to-benefit ratio is convincingly in favor of this postoperative pain relief strategy (Nimmo, 2004).

Reports from centers where epidural analgesia is currently used in major abdominal surgery patients and effectively supervised by acute pain service personnel have shown a complication rate similar to that described for other forms of analgesia (McLeod et al.,2001;

Nimmo, 2004; Rigg et al., 2002). In order to decrease the incidence of potentially severe complications, the candidates to epidural analgesia must be carefully selected. In this context, the technique should be avoided in septic subjects and those bearing coagulation disorders.

Several, less severe cardio-respiratory disturbances are straightly related to the administration of analgesic regimen into the epidural space. Thus, mild hypotension and bradycardia are well-recognized hemodynamic consequences of epidural induced sympatholysis, that could be balanced by fluid administration (Moraca et al., 2003). In patients with cardiopulmonary pathology in which postoperative fluid overload is undesirable, vasopressors represent the preferred treatment for hypotension, since both ephedrine and fluids have demonstrated comparable hemodynamic effects (Waurick & Van Aken, 2004).

The opioid-induced respiratory dysfunction has an incidence estimated to be less than 10% comparable to systemic opioids (Moraca et al., 2003). The use of combination of local anesthetic and opioid on epidural route reduces the amount of opioid needed and thus the risk of its subsequent effect of respiratory depression (Moraca et al., 2003; Nimmo, 2004).

Systemic absorption of local anesthetic at high doses can produce seizures, coma and cardiac arrhythmias, the magnitude of such toxicity reactions being related to the type and concentration of anesthetic (Moraca et al., 2003).

Other potential problems with epidural analgesia are related to catheter placement and removal. Accidental dural puncture during needle insertion has been found in 0.16-1.3% in a series of 51.000 epidural catheters (Moraca et al., 2003).

Neurovascular damage during catheter insertion is uncommon too (Moraca et al., 2003). Thus, transient neurologic symptoms represented by sharp radicular back pain or paresthesias due to nerve root irritation by the catheter simply resolve after its removal (Moraca et al., 2003).

Injury to the spinal vasculature during catheter insertion or removal, described in approximately 3-12% of cases could rarely transform into symptomatic epidural hematoma. The incidence of epidural hematoma has been estimated to be less than 1 in 150.000 in one study, and respectively none in another series of 100.000 (Moraca et al., 2003). On the other hand, it is well demonstrated that symptomatic epidural hematomas are associated with the use of anticoagulant therapy, catheter placement or removal during anticoagulation or trauma during catheter insertion (Moraca et al., 2003).

The use of anticoagulation and the risk of epidural hematoma formation in subjects receiving epidural analgesia has been a controversial issue. Despite this debate, safety of both therapeutic anticoagulation and deep venous thrombosis prophylaxis in patients with postoperative epidural analgesia has been reported in multiple studies (Moraca et al., 2003). In any case, the risk of bleeding complications should be cautiously evaluated in balance with the potential benefits of epidural analgesia on an individual basis.

Catheter-related infections, namely meningitis and epidural abscess are rare (Moraca at al., 2003). Retaining epidural catheter in situ longer than 3 days and nonsterile technique increase the risk of these complications that lead to potentially devastating neurological disturbances. Early recognition of neurological disturbances that may herald an epidural hematoma or abscess completed with immediate imaging investigations and decompressive laminectomy within 8 hours of diagnosis have shown to improve neurologic prognosis (Nimmo, 2004).

Taking into account that epidural analgesia carries certain risks, despite objective improvements in outcome, in major abdominal surgery patients, vigilant monitoring during early postoperative period has to be guaranteed (Nimmo, 2004).

In other terms, modern analgesic practice inherently safe, together with professional surveillance during postoperative period could minimize the risk of potential complications, thus improving major abdominal surgery outcomes and patient satisfaction.

5. Integration of postoperative epidural analgesia into rehabilitation program

In recent years, extensive data have demonstrated positive physiological effects of postoperative epidural analgesia on several organ systems in major abdominal surgery patients (Kehlet, 2008). It is therefore surprising that the overall progress registered with this pain relieving technique in terms of postoperative morbidity has been limited, sometimes even non-demonstrable by clinical trials (Kehlet & Holte, 2001). The most plausible explanation is that a single-modality intervention, namely effective pain relief, for a complex problem such as postoperative morbidity will provide few improvements in outcome (Kehlet, 2008; Kehlet & Holte, 2001).

A multimodal approach consisting into a complex postoperative rehabilitation program seems to be more rational. The postoperative care package involves mainly four factors: effective epidural analgesia, as an essential part but not the only one, limiting the stress response to surgery, early mobilization and oral nutrition (Kehlet, 2008; Kehlet & Wilmore, 2008; Nimmo, 2004).

The use of well-documented physiological advantages of epidural analgesia in such a postoperative care program leads to decrease of morbidity across major abdominal procedures and significantly improves the quality of postoperative recovery (Kehlet, 2008; Kehlet & Wilmore, 2008).

Findings of many clinical trials are relevant in this respect. Thus, patients with major abdominal procedures managed in a multimodal care program including epidural analgesia have demonstrated earlier discharge from intensive-care unit, earlier return of normal bowel function, reduced catabolism and less fatigue than those undergoing equivalent surgery but not participating in such a postoperative care program (Carli et al., 2002; Kehlet, 2008; Nimmo, 2004).

A successful multimodal rehabilitation program requires the reorganization of traditional acute pain service activity, with emphasis on functional recovery (Kehlet & Holte, 2001). Increased collaborative effort of the patient, anesthetist, surgeon and surgical nurse undoubtedly improves the rate of progress in postoperative outcome. The revision of traditional postoperative care program with drains, gastrointestinal tubes, catheters, prolonged fasting and other restrictions is mandatory, too (Kehlet & Holte, 2001).

Educational programs have to be developed in order to analyze postoperative pathophysiology, as well as the factors that could limit early recovery after each individual major abdominal procedure (Kehlet & Dahl, 2003; Kehlet & Wilmore, 2008).

A key element for multimodal rehabilitation program is the implementation and development of daily nurse care programs that could improve the quality of postoperative care, thus facilitating early recovery after major abdominal procedures (Kehlet & Holte, 2001).

The concept of multimodal postoperative rehabilitation program with epidural analgesia as a key factor, that provides effective control of postoperative pain after major abdominal surgery allowing early mobilization and oral feeding, together with the stress-reducing effect, has gained acceptance of patients, acute pain practitioners and surgeons, being the single strategy that could significantly improve postoperative outcome.

6. Conclusions and future directions for research

One of the main issues of concern to patients presenting for major abdominal surgery is postoperative analgesia. Consequently, provision of high-quality postoperative pain control remains an important goal for acute pain service activity.

Epidural analgesia is considered as the gold standard analgesic technique for major abdominal procedures. This strategy has the potential to provide complete analgesia and it is particularly effective at optimizing functional pain relief, thus improving patient satisfaction and postoperative outcome.

There is consistent evidence that epidural analgesia in major abdominal surgery has positive physiological effects on cardiovascular and pulmonary functions, paralytic ileus and catabolism, all of which theoretically leading to reduced major morbidity and mortality.

The accuracy of this finding should become irrelevant because of contemporary changes in medical practice with rapid conversion of major abdominal surgery to laparoscopic procedures and implementation of fast-track programs.

A critical limitation of nearly all discussed studies is the relatively small number of patients that have been enrolled. The low incidence of postoperative complications and reduced rate of mortality require increasingly large randomized clinical trials and the acquisition of large amounts of patient data.

The concept of multimodal rehabilitation program in which epidural analgesia is a key component represents a major task. The potential positive effects of epidural analgesia on postoperative outcome might not live up to expectations unless these physiological advantages are used in the multimodal postoperative rehabilitation program. The other therapeutic factors (early mobilization, early oral nutrition, fluid balance) must be integrated into future studies examining postoperative outcome after major abdominal surgery.

With safety modern anesthetic practice and minimally invasive surgical techniques it is the time to increase the scope of definition of outcomes of interest. As mortality and major morbidity become uncommon, even in high-risk abdominal procedures, the future studies may need to focus on patient's own views of recovery. These nontraditional outcomes assessed from the patient's perspective comprise quality of postoperative recovery including analgesia, well being state, return to preoperative energy and activity level and quality of life.

Epidural analgesia is time-consuming, it requires specific technical skills and pharmacological abilities and professional surveillance. Clearly, epidural analgesia is not devoid of risks and failures may occur.

Our analysis provide an evidence base for rational decision making to help the anesthesiologist in choosing the most beneficial use of epidurals in major abdominal surgery patients.

7. References

Agnelli, G. (2004). Prevention of venous thromboembolism in surgical patients. *Circulation*, Vol. 110, No. 24, Suppl. IV, (December 2004), pp. 4-12, ISSN: 1524-4539

Ballantyne, J.; Carr, D. & deFerranti, S. (1998). The comparative effects of postoperative analgesic therapies on pulmonary outcome: Cumulative meta-analyses of randomized, controlled trials. *Anesthesia & Analgesia*, Vol. 86, No. 3, (March 1998), pp. 598-612, ISSN 1526-7598

Bartha, E.; Carlsson, P. & Kalman, S. (2006). Evaluation of costs and effects of epidural analgesia and patient-controlled intravenous analgesia after major abdominal surgery. *British Journal of Anaesthesia*, Vol. 96, No. 1, (January 2006), pp. 111-117, ISSN 1471-6771

Basse, L.; Hjort, J. & Billesbølle, P. (2000). A clinical pathway to accelerate recovery after colonic resection. *Annals of Surgery*, Vol. 232, No. 1, (July 2000), pp. 51-57, ISSN 1528-1140

Bauer, A. & Boeckxstaens, G. (2004). Mechanisms of postoperative ileus. *Neurogastroenterology & Motility*, Vol. 16, Issue Supplement s2, (October 2004), pp. 54-60

Beattie, S.; Badner, N. & Choi, P. (2001). Epidural analgesia reduces postoperative myocardial infarction: A meta-analysis. *Anesthesia & Analgesia*, Vol. 93, No. 4, (October 2001), pp. 853-858, ISSN 1526-7598

Beilin, B.; Shavit, Y. & Trabekin, E. (2003). The effects of postoperative pain management on immune response to surgery. *Anesthesia & Analgesia*, Vol. 97, No. 3, (September 2003), pp. 822-827, ISSN 1526-7598

Block, B.; Liu, S. & Rowlingson, A. (2003). Efficacy of postoperative epidural analgesia: A meta-analysis. *The Journal of the American Medical Association*, Vol. 290, No. 18, (November 2003), pp. 2455-2463, ISSN: 1538-3598

Bombeli, T. & Spahn, D. (2004). Updates in perioperative coagulation: Physiology and management of thromboembolism and haemorrhage. *British Journal of Anaesthesia*, Vol. 93, No. 2, (August 2004), pp. 275-287, ISSN 1471-6771

Carli, F.; Mayo, N. & Klubien, K. (2002). Epidural analgesia enhances functional exercise capacity and health-related quality of life after colonic surgery: results of a randomized trial. *Anesthesiology*, Vol.97, No. 3, (September 2002), pp. 540-549, ISSN 0003-3022

Devereaux, P.; Goldman, L. & Cook, D. (2005). Perioperative cardiac events in patients undergoing noncardiac surgery: A review of the magnitude of the problem, the pathophysiology of the events and methods to estimate and communicate risk. *Canadian Medical Association Journal*, Vol. 173, No. 6, (September 2005), pp. 627-634, ISSN 1488-2329

Dolin, S.; Cashman, J. & Bland, J. (2002). Effectiveness of acute postoperative pain management: I. Evidence from published data. *British Journal of Anaesthesia*, Vol. 89, No. 3, (September 2002), pp. 409-423, ISSN 1471-6771

Fong, H.; Sands, L. & Leung, J. (2006). The role of postoperative analgesia in delirium and cognitive decline in elderly patients: A systematic review. *Anesthesia & Analgesia*, Vol. 102, No. 4, (April 2006), pp. 1255-1266, ISSN 1526-7598

Grass, J. (2000). The role of epidural anesthesia and analgesia in postoperative outcome. *Anesthesiology Clinics of North America*, Vol. 18, No. 2, (June 2000), pp. 407-428

Groeben, H.; Schäfer, B. & Pavlakovic, G. (2002). Lung function under high thoracic segmental epidural anesthesia with ropivacaine or bupivacaine in patients with severe obstructive pulmonary disease undergoing breast surgery. *Anesthesiology*, Vol. 96, No. 3, (March 2002), pp. 536-541, ISSN 0003-3022

Gruber, E.; Tschernko, E. & Kritzinger, M. (2001). The effects of thoracic epidural analgesia with bupivacaine 0.25% on ventilatory mechanics in patients with severe chronic obstructive pulmonary disease. *Anesthesia & Analgesia*, Vol. 92, No. 4, (April 2001), pp. 1015-1019, ISSN 1526-7598

Holte, K. & Kehlet, H. (2002). Epidural anaesthesia and analgesia – effects on surgical stress responses and implications for postoperative nutrition. *Clinical Nutrition*, Vol. 21, No. 3, (June 2002), pp. 199-206, ISSN 0261-5614

Jiang, S.; Li, Z. & Huang, L. (2005). Multivariate analysis of the risk for pulmonary complication after gastrointestinal surgery. *World Journal of Gastroenterology*, Vol. 11, No. 24, (June 2005), pp. 3735-3741, ISSN 1007-9327

Jørgensen, H.; Wetterslev, J. & Møiniche, S. (2000). Epidural local anaesthetics versus opioid-based analgesic regimens on postoperative gastrointestinal paralysis, PONV and pain after abdominal surgery. In: *Cochrane Database of Systematic Reviews 2001*, 23.10.2000, Available from http://www2.cochrane.org/reviews/en/ab001893.html

Kabon, B.; Fleischmann, E. & Treschan, T. (2003). Thoracic epidural anesthesia increases tissue oxygenation during major abdominal surgery. *Anesthesia & Analgesia*, Vol. 97, No. 6, (December 2003), pp. 1812-1816, ISSN 1526-7598

Kehlet, H. (1994). Postoperative pain relief—what is the issue? *British Journal of Anaesthesia*, Vol. 72, No. 4, (April 1994), pp. 375-378, ISSN 1471-6771

Kehlet, H. (1997). Multimodal approach to control postoperative pathophysiology and rehabilitation. *British Journal of Anaesthesia*, Vol. 78, No. 5, (May 1997), pp. 606-617, ISSN 1471-6771

Kehlet, H. & Holte, K. (2001). Effect of postoperative analgesia on surgical outcome. *British Journal of Anaesthesia*, Vol. 87, No. 1, (June 2001), pp. 62-72, ISSN 1471-6771

Kehlet, H. & Dahl, J. (2003). Anaesthesia, surgery and challenges in postoperative recovery. *The Lancet*, Vol. 362, No. 9399, (December 2003), pp. 1921-1928

Kehlet, H. (2008). Fast-track colorectal surgery. *The Lancet*, Vol. 371, No. 9615, (March 2008), pp. 791-793

Kehlet, H. & Wilmore, D. (2008). Evidence-based surgical care and the evolution of fast-track surgery. *Annals of Surgery*, Vol. 248, No. 2, (August 2008), pp. 189-198, ISSN 1528-1140

Liu, S. & Wu, C. (2007). Effect of postoperative analgesia on major postoperative complications: A systemic update of the evidence. *Anesthesia & Analgesia*, Vol. 104, No. 3, (March 2007), pp. 689-702, ISSN 1526-7598

Nigärd, E.; Kofoed, K. & Freiberg, J. (2005). Effects of high thoracic epidural analgesia on myocardial blood flow in patients with ischemic heart disease. *Circulation*, Vol. 111, No. 17, (May 2005), pp. 2165-2170, ISSN: 1524-4539

Nimmo, S. (2004). Benefit and outcome after epidural analgesia. *Continuing Education in Anaesthesia, Critical Care & Pain*, Vol. 4, No. 2, (April 2004), pp. 44-47, ISSN 1743-1824

McLeod, G.; Davies, H. & Munnoch N. (2001). Postoperative pain relief using thoracic epidural analgesia: Outstanding success and disappointing failures. *Anaesthesia*, Vol. 56, No. 1, (January 2001), pp. 75-81

Moraca, R.; Sheldon, D. & Thirlby, R. (2003). The role of epidural anesthesia and analgesia in surgical practice. *Annals of Surgery*, Vol. 238, No. 5, (November 2003), pp. 663-673, ISSN 1528-1140

Mythen, M. (2005). Postoperative gastrointestinal tract dysfunction. *Anesthesia & Analgesia*, Vol. 100, No. 1, (January 2005), pp. 196-204, ISSN 1526-7598

Park, W.; Thompson, J. & Lee, K. (2001). Effect of epidural anesthesia and analgesia on perioperative outcome: A randomized, controlled veterans affairs cooperative study. *Annals of Surgery*, Vol. 234, No. 4, (October 2001), pp. 560-571, ISSN 1528-1140

Paulsen, E.; Porter, M. & Helmer, S. (2001). Thoracic epidural versus patient-controlled analgesia in elective bowel resections. *The American Journal of Surgery*, Vol. 182, No. 6, (December 2001), pp. 570-577, ISSN 0002-9610

Peyton, P.; Myles, P. & Silbert, B. (2003). Perioperative epidural analgesia and outcome after major abdominal surgery in high-risk patients. *Anesthesia & Analgesia*, Vol. 96, No. 2, (February 2003), pp. 548-554, ISSN 1526-7598

Pöpping, D.; Elia, N. & Marret, E. (2008). Protective effects of epidural analgesia on pulmonary complications after abdominal and thoracic surgery. *Archives of Surgery*, Vol. 143, No. 10, (October 2008), pp. 990-999

Rigg, J.; Jamrozik, K. & Myles, P. (2000). Design of the multicenter Australian study of epidural anesthesia and analgesia in major surgery: The MASTER trial. *Controlled Clinical Trials*, Vol. 21, No. 3, (June 2000), pp. 244-256

Rigg, J.; Jamrozik, K. & Myles, P. (2002). Epidural anaesthesia and analgesia an outcome of major surgery: A randomized trial. *The Lancet*, Vol. 359, No. 9314, (April 2002), pp. 1276-1282

Roderick, P.; Ferris, G. & Wilson, K. (2005). Towards evidence-based guidelines for the prevention of venous thromboembolism: Systematic reviews of mechanical methods, oral anticoagulation, dextran and regional anaesthesia as thromboprophylaxis. *Health Technology Assessment*, Vol. 9, No. 49, (December 2005), pp. 1-94

Sido, B.; Teklote, J. & Hartel, M. (2004). Inflammatory response after abdominal surgery. *Best Practice & Research: Clinical Anaesthesiology*, Vol. 18, No. 3, (September 2004), pp. 439-454, ISSN 1521-6896

Warner, D. (2000). Preventing postoperative pulmonary complications: the role of anesthesiologist. *Anesthesiology*, Vol. 92, No. 5, (May 2000), pp.1467-1472, ISSN 0003-3022

Waurick, R. & Van Aken, H. (2005). Update in thoracic epidural anaesthesia. *Best Practice & Research: Clinical Anaesthesiology*, Vol. 19, No. 2, (June 2005), pp.201-213, ISSN 1521-6896

Werawatganon, T. & Charuluxananan, S. (2005). Patient controlled intravenous opioid analgesia versus continuous epidural analgesia for pain after intra-abdominal surgery. *Anesthesia & Analgesia*, Vol. 100, No. 5, (May 2005), pp. 1536, ISSN 1526-7598

Wheatley, R.; Shug, S. & Watson, D. (2001). Safety and efficacy of postoperative epidural analgesia. *British Journal of Anaesthesia*, Vol. 87, No. 1, (June 2001), pp. 47-61, ISSN 1471-6771

Wu, C.; Cohen, S. & Richman, J. (2005). Efficacy of postoperative patient-controlled and continuous infusion epidural analgesia versus intravenous patient-controlled analgesia with opioids: A meta-analysis. *Anesthesiology*, Vol. 103, No. 5, (November 2005), pp. 1079-1088, ISSN 0003-3022

Yokoyama, M.; Itano, Y. & Katayama, H. (2005). The effects of continuous epidural anesthesia and analgesia on stress response and immune function in patients undergoing radical esophagectomy. *Anesthesia & Analgesia*, Vol. 101, No. 5, (November 2005), pp. 1521-1527, ISSN 1526-7598

6

Epidural Analgesia in Labour from a Sociological Perspective – A Case Analysis of Andalusia, Spain

Rafael Serrano-del-Rosal,
Lourdes Biedma-Velázquez and José Mª García-de-Diego
Institute for Advanced Social Studies,
Spanish National Research Council (IESA/CSIC), Córdoba
Spain

1. Introduction

Health is a key area for humans and the main indicator of the quality of life we enjoy. For this reason health has been studied, analysed, and discussed across numerous scientific disciplines from a wide range of theoretical perspectives. From the quantitative point of view, it is noteworthy that life expectancy in Western countries has reached its highest level in the history of mankind[1]. Medical research has made significant contributions to our understanding of the human organism, as well as the treatment and prevention of many diseases. These advances have had a direct impact not only on increased life expectancy, but have also changed the concept of medical practice, which is increasingly focused on "adding life to years rather than adding years to life" (Herrera & Duran, 1995). Indeed, in medical practice today, the patient's quality of life has become as or even more important than the disease itself. From the qualitative standpoint, this has led to a significant change in how health is conceived. Health is now understood as a multidimensional concept that in addition to purely medical aspects (morbidity, mortality, life expectancy), encompasses physical elements (physical surrounding, housing, the environment, etc.), social components (occupational health and safety, education and health care, equitable distribution of available resources, etc.), lifestyle (adequate diet, physical exercise, tobacco and alcohol consumption, etc.), the healthcare system (physical and human resources, hospital care, social security, research, etc.), and others.

The health as a multidimensional concept where the culture and society to which an individual belongs, alongside its norms, values and roles, influence they way that individuals experience health problems, condition such experiences even when they are not the cause of the illness or disease itself, and affect how individuals deal with them. Similarly, at the political level, institutions, organisations, and the entire fabric of a

---

[1] According to data from 2004 for Spain, the life expectancy at birth was 77 years for men and 83 years for women (Source: WHO)

government influence how a health "problem" is viewed, financed, legitimised or delegitimised (Cockerham, 2002).

For this reason, sociology has now been incorporated into health analyses and the interpretation of medical events. Sociology contributes to the medical discipline by analysing the social causes and consequences of health and disease in individuals. It therefore goes beyond integrating a subjective approach to medical events, but encompasses a global social vision.

From the sociological perspective, health cannot be understood as a purely biological event involving physical and chemical elements. As the World Health Organization (WHO) has acknowledged, the concept of health goes beyond the purely biomedical and is a state of complete physical, mental, and social well-being and not merely the absence of disease or infirmity (WHO, 1952). Indeed, it is precisely these social elements affecting health and disease that is of concern to the field of sociology.

One issue of particular interest to sociological research in this sphere is the analysis of social inequalities in health. The existence of health disparities have been reported for most countries of the world (Starfield, 2002), with the most disadvantaged, women, and immigrants from low-income countries showing the worse health indicators.

This field of study examines, for example, inequalities due to gender, that is, the social condition of being male or female and not the biological bases characterising gender. It has been shown (Rohfs et al., 2000) that although women generally have lower mortality rates and a longer life expectancy, they also suffer from more chronic diseases, have higher levels of disability, suffer more pain, respond more poorly to analgesics, and report more negative perceptions about their own health. Some researchers attribute differences in health to biological and genetic variations (Mogil, 2004; Greenspan et al., 2007), while others point to the psychological and social components of these differences (Hanna et al., 2009; Breivik et al., 2006). However, scholars are unable to explain all the differences, nor do all the studies have a solely biological basis.

In this chapter we analyse health as a social concept, focusing specifically on the role of women in medicine as subjective and passive elements of medical practice. This approach will serve as the basis of our analysis of the use of epidural analgesia during childbirth, which is explored in the second part of the chapter. In the first part we deal with pain as a social element and provide an overview of the history of pain and the evolution of treatment for pain.

2. Pain as a social element

Pain, like health and illness, is the representation of an individual state that is only possible for "others" to decipher through the patient's own perception of suffering (Baszanger, 1992). According to this approach, pain is defined, in addition to its physical, biological and chemical components, according to the norms, values and symbols that the sick or ailing, those who accompany them, and the health professionals who care for them attach to such pain. In other words, pain is defined according to the social meaning conferred to it.

But pain has not always been interpreted in the same manner. Therefore, in this section we first attempt to contextualise pain as a social element. We then go on to provide a brief overview of how pain has been interpreted socially throughout history, and finally discuss the use and extent of anesthesia and analgesics to relieve pain.

2.1 Conceptualisation of pain as a social elements

Pain has accompanied human beings throughout history (Pérez-Cajaraville et al., 2005), but has not always been interpreted the same way (Le Breton, 1999, 2010). The manner in which pain is interpreted has changed as have society and culture, which have attempted to convey meaning to pain. Pain is a disruptive experience that forces individuals to seek meaning for the ailments they suffer from (Barragán-Solís, 2006).

Pain has an undeniable physical and anatomical component (Loeser & Melzack, 1999), as well as a cultural and social component, which lead it to be interpreted from different perspectives (Kirmayer, 2008). Yet the social component of pain has not always been taken into account and was, for a long time, treated merely as a sign that something physical or organic was not functioning properly.

Today, however, the multidimensionality of pain has been widely accepted. The International Association for the Study of Pain (IASP) defines pain as an unpleasant sensory (objective) and emotional (subjective) experience associated with actual (injury) or potential (pathology) tissue damage, or described in terms of such damage (as if it already existed and were the cause) (IASP, 1979; Guevara-López, 2004).

Nowadays it is much more difficult to define pain as it is viewed as a somatic sensation (Franco, 1999) that can only be determined through the personal interpretation of the patient who "lives" the painful experience (Leriche, 1937), that is, according to the subjective perception of the individual (Suvin et al., 2005). Moreover, data from studies that have attempted to "objectively" measure pain have been largely unsatisfactory. From a sociological perspective, pain is conditioned not only by the particular elements characterising the sufferer, that is, the subjective view of pain or what has been called "private pain" (Mosoco, 2002), but also by social elements or "public pain" that affect the sufferer such as education, culture, society, politics, and others.

The fact that people with less educational level have been found to suffer more pain than those with a higher level cannot be explained by biological factors, but rather as a set of social effects that have had an influence on the occurrence of the event. To reduce these inequalities it is therefore necessary to determine which elements are most relevant in explaining social inequalities in health.

However, pain as a process for which individuals seek meaning cannot be removed from the actual cause of the pain. Chronic pain due to an incapacitating disease is not perceived in the same manner as an occasional sharp pain that is not severely inhabilitating and can be overcome with a more or less rapid cure (Biedma-Velázquez et al., 2010). This second context refers to pain during childbirth and occasional, transitory pain, which is the result of a biological event that does not constitute an illness, usually has a positive outcome (a birth), and for which there is no fear of future renewal or intensification (Bayes, 1998); all of which affect the perception of pain. However, pain during labour is very intense (Fernandez & Villalonga, 2000) and greater than that experienced by other animal species. To this we must add elements such as fear, anxiety and stress that can increase pain and make labour difficult (Calderon et al, 2006). Such factors have prompted the search for methods to alleviate the suffering of mothers during childbirth. Indeed, in this quest to eliminate pain, physicians in particular and the medical discipline in general are currently responsible for putting an end to and managing pain in today's society.

2.2 History of pain and its social interpretation

Although pain and disease have accompanied humans throughout history, they have not always been interpreted in the same manner. In this chapter we will obviously not attempt to provide a comprehensive overview on the history of pain as excellent reviews on pain already exist. However, we would like to highlight different conceptions of pain with a view to understanding how the culture and society to which an individual belongs condition the way pain is experienced. To do so, we rely chiefly on the work of Bonica, 1990; Morris, 1991; Perez-Cajaraville et al., 2005; Perez et al., 2005; and Krivoy et al., 2010.

Primitive peoples believed that pain was caused by demons or spirits entering bodily orifices. Given that these primitive societies did not make a distinction between the spirit and the body, tribal shamans and sorcerers played a dual role as both priests of the spirit and healers of the body. Moreover, in these cultures pain was considered a rite of passage; something that was not only inevitable but desirable and sought after as a passage to adulthood, social prestige or a new status.

This concept of pain persisted among primitive tribes for a long time, especially in ancient Native American cultures, or other primitive tribes throughout several periods in history. The notion that pain entered bodily orifices was common in ancient Egypt, albeit the Egyptians made considerable advances in this regard such as the development of a body of medical professionals grouped into specialised schools overseen by priests.

The notion that pain comes from an outside source and is something external to man as a means to pass a test or as punishment has persisted throughout much of humanity to a greater or lesser degree. In Judeo-Christian culture, pain was considered the manifestation of divine punishment for man's sin. The Old Testament contains numerous references to pain as being synonymous with sin, as punishment for humanity's ills or as evidence of man's loyalty to God (Jaron, 1991). Part of this concept of pain was reflected in the New Testament and medieval Europe, permeating traditions, customs and conceptions of health and illness that have survived until today.

Buddhism views pain as a form of punishment for a sin committed in this or a previous life, although it introduces an innovative element of great importance: the psychological component of pain.

The Greeks, particularly Hippocrates and later his disciples, did not reject the role of the gods in pain, but also began to seek a more pragmatic meaning for pain by considering it a sign that something in the body was not functioning properly, thus providing a biological explanation for the process of pain. This view of pain as a "symptom" has endured and constituted an important turning point in the evolution of medicine.

From this moment onwards, explanations for pain sought its origin in different parts of the human organism. Aristotle taught that pain originated in the heart alongside feelings, and considered pain a "disease of the soul". Later, Galen and others, believed that pain originated in the brain, dissociating it from the supernatural, and opening the door to the role of the nervous system and neurons in pain. Nevertheless, whether in the heart or the brain, pain remains a symptom that something is wrong.

During the Middle Ages, pain was again interpreted in Europe according to the philosophical teachings of Aristotle and strongly influenced by religious thought, mainly Christian doctrine. These doctrines legitimised suffering and pain as a way of approaching God; a way to atone for past, present or future sins; and an element of purification and redemption. According to this notion, which went so far as to promote martyrdom, combating pain was considered a negative and "unnatural" behaviour. In particular, pain during childbirth was considered the "price" that women had to pay for being the cause of man's exile from paradise, and according to the Old Testament, as a "gift" that women must learn to appreciate.

It was not until the Renaissance that the classic texts reopened the debate on the origin, treatment and interpretation of pain due to a renewed interest in the scientific knowledge of medicine. At the time, science and religion lived side-by-side in a tense equilibrium in which religion served to explain the source of pain, while science dictated how to combat it. Once again, pain was regarded as a symptom that something was not quite right.

The eighteenth century was a time of great scientific and theoretical advances in the fields of anatomy, physics and chemistry. Medicine was gradually moving away from religion; a retreat that was more marked in subsequent centuries until the two ultimately separated in the twentieth century.

The twentieth century brought other substantial and important changes. One was the more or less formal inclusion of psychological elements in the definition of pain. After treating a large number of wounded soldiers during World War II, Dr. Beecher observed the effect of "placebo" drugs on pain, finding that the mind played a key role in the perception of pain. Indeed, pain could no longer be explained merely as a symptom, but as a reflection of something else; a suffering that is not always related to a biological problem. Leriche (1937), a pioneer in the treatment of surgical pain, is another important reference in twentieth century medicine. Had pain not been controlled in surgery, many of the common and everyday operations performed today would not have been possible. Thanks to Leriche's contributions, medicine has made significant advances regarding pain relief.

Dr. Bonica (1953) established the world's first multidisciplinary pain clinic. His concern, vision and understanding of pain laid the grounds for a model to manage pain that continues to be emulated to this day and opened the door to the first professionals specialised in pain management.

The late twentieth and early twenty-first century could be defined as the culture of disease prevention and medicalisation. Enormous advances have been made in biomedical research in the West and medical interventions are now performed that were unthinkable just a century ago. The use of anesthesia and analgesics have now become common place under the philosophy that pain is in many ways useless, sterile and demeaning (Le Breton, 1999). As a consequence, the social threshold regarding the tolerance of pain has decreased.

Today, pain is no longer viewed merely as a sign or symptom that something is wrong, but has begun to be perceived as a disease in itself. The idea that pain functions as an alarm is beginning to lose force, while patients increasingly request to live with as little pain as possible. Traditional medicine has given way to a new "patient-centred" medicine (Baszanger, 1992) in which patients have the say and physicians must try to address their needs. As occurred in the past with priests, the hegemony that physicians enjoyed as experts has now been lost to some extent.

2.3 Treatment of pain

It should come as no surprise that the treatment of pain has been conditioned by the very concept and meaning attributed to pain. Thus, for example, if one considers that pain is not only natural but even "good", either because it brings us closer to God, or because it is a symptom, a clue that "something is wrong" and helps us diagnose the real disease, eliminating pain will not only not be a priority, but could be considered an error.

How pain is treated is also influenced by the role of the patient, and how the patient manifests his or her pain. Depending on whether or not a patient feels they have the right to express their pain or on how the disease is perceived by society, it will be more or less socially acceptable to attempt to alleviate pain caused by disease. Drugs and treatments for pain are also subject to social evaluation. If one believes that a certain drug or treatment is useful in alleviating pain, the treatment is more likely to be effective than when the treatment is discredited or its effectiveness is questioned by society. For these reasons pain relief treatments are also the object of social research since they are, at one and the same time, a reflection and a cause of the society in which they arise or are developed.

While pain is as old as mankind, so are the attempts to alleviate it. From the shamans of ancient primitive communities to today's pain clinics, the search for ways to free human beings from the suffering caused by acute or chronic pain have continued to evolve. Pain during labour and delivery is no exception, and has been the objective of various techniques and methods to minimise or eliminate pain during childbirth.

We have knowledge of the use of medicinal plants by primitive peoples as early as 4000 BC. These societies believed that pain and sickness were gods' way of punishing man. Because diseases and illnesses were thought to enter through the body's orifices, treatments for pain responded to this conception. For this reason, tribal priests, shamans and sorcerers were responsible for relieving pain, curing members of the tribe and acting as mediators with the spiritual world. They also performed complex practices such as trepanation as a way of freeing spirits and ridding the ill and ailing of pain.

There are many references to the different medicinal uses of many plants throughout the history of mankind. We know that hashish was employed as anesthesia in ancient China and that opium was used in Greece as a means "to forget one's sorrows" (Morris, 1991). The use of white willow bark (a predecessor of acetylsalicylic acid) has also been documented to relieve labour pain.

When pain is related to coming closer to God, as was common in the Middle Ages, the ailing resort to God, saints virgins, penance and atonement for sins rather than medicine to alleviate pain. The church rejected the use of analgesics and other drugs as many medical practices were believed to be the work of Satan and "evil". Nonetheless, drugs and anesthetics were used, but mainly under the tutelage of the church, which had its own body of physician-priests who decided which medical practices were allowed in accordance with Christian faith and which were not.

The Renaissance was a time of greater tolerance and permitted the use of medications forgotten during the Middle Ages. In the eighteenth century, the advent of modern anesthesia and pharmacology marked a turning point in the treatment of pain.

The nineteenth century saw the birth of ether and morphine, great allies in the fight against pain. In fact, James and Simpson (1847) introduced the use of ether as an anaesthetic during labour (Pérez-Cajaraville et al., 2005) despite the conservative currents of thought of the time which believed that women should suffer during childbirth, as God wills. The divide between medicine and religion gradually widened until the twentieth century when a clear distinction was made between both.

As described above, today the focus has turned to preventing pain. Enormous advances have been made in the treatment and relief of pain, the development of anaesthetic methods and the establishment of pain clinics.

Until recently, midwives played a predominant role in the childbirth process, while gynecologists and obstetricians remained in the background (Campuzano, 2007) in the event of complications. Childbirth was considered a "natural" event that did not require medical supervision; and just as natural as the fact of being born, was the fact that women were expected to suffer pain during the process.

As epidural analgesia came to be used more widely in childbirths in Spain in the 1990s (Torres, 1999), the role of physicians and anaesthesiologists underwent enormous changes. They once again came to play an important role in the process, with both organisations and personnel having to adapt to these new changes.

3. Supply of obstetric epidural analgesia

Today, epidural analgesia is the most widely used method of pain relief in childbirth. This does not mean that the method is free of complications or contraindications, but these are considered to be of minor importance and a generally infrequent event. In general, the gains outweigh the losses and epidurals are now regarded as a safe method for both mothers and babies (Torres A, 1999; De la Torre & Pérez-Iraola, 2002, Fernández-Guisaola et al., 2004) provided there are no specific medical indications that advise against or prevent using this anesthesia and informed consent has been obtained from the expectant mother. However, each case must be analysed individually by trained and qualified professionals.

3.1 The implementation of obstetric epidural analgesia in Spanish hospitals

As mentioned above, drugs to relieve pain in childbirth have a long history of use. The first lumbar epidural analgesia technique was described in 1921 (Pagés, F, 1921), but the technique would not begin to be employed until the late sixties (Fernández-Guisasola, 2003). Spain, however, would have to wait until the 1980s before epidural analgesia came to be used, mainly in private hospitals. By the 1990s there was a spectacular increase in the demand for epidural analgesia, which was introduced into many public hospitals (Fernández-Guisasola, 2003).

The provision of epidural analgesia in Spain was largely the result of a report of great impact known as the *Plan Integral de la Atención a la Mujer* (Comprehensive Plan for the Care of Women, 1998). Following the publication of the report, epidural analgesia was offered to all pregnant women in Spanish hospitals in 2000.

Today, women in Spain are ensured a series of rights during labour and delivery by law (Law 41/2002). Specifically, they are entitled to be informed about all aspects of the clinical care they receive during childbirth; and the information they are given must be easy to understand, appropriate to their needs, and aid them in making decisions freely. Once informed, women have the right to decide about their own health and body and to refuse any treatment or clinical intervention that is proposed to them. They have the right to choose freely from among the available clinical options including the birthing position, continuous or intermittent monitoring, the possibility of walking or remain lying down during labour, whether they want to receive epidural analgesia or not, or receive constant emotional support during delivery. The ability to choose is only limited by the availability of options, that is, the services provided at each hospital.

In this regard, the law has elevated epidural analgesia during childbirth to the category of a right. As in other neighbouring countries, before a woman gives birth in a hospital in Andalusia in particular, and in Spain in general, they must be provided the so-called "*Plan de Parto*" or Birth Plan, which in addition to informing them about the birthing process, also provides information on epidural analgesia and asks women to decide whether or not to use it.

But introducing epidural analgesia in Spanish hospitals has not been an easy task. Not only have hospitals not developed the necessary infrastructure at the same pace, but it has also been necessary to train professionals in the protocol of this technique (Campuzano, 2007).

However, according to the General Law of Health (Law 14/1986), "public health care will be extended to the entire Spanish population" and "access and health care will be provided in conditions of effective equality" to prevent discrimination for territorial, social, or other reasons. To achieve this aim, a common portfolio of specialised care services was developed for the entire country (Royal Decree 1030/2006). This portfolio includes the use of epidural analgesia according to health service protocols for so-called "normal" pregnancies.

To promote the widespread use of epidural analgesia in Spain, the health agencies of the autonomous communities regulated the use of this method in the 1990s. In this regard, Andalusia has been a pioneering region (Decree 101/1995). However, in spite of these legislative regulations, the use of epidurals was not implemented in an equal manner or at the same rate in all the hospitals of Andalusia, prompting complaints from users. Indeed, citizens claimed their right to health protection, which not only encompasses health care in the event of a disease or illness, but also care to alleviate pain as in the case of labour and delivery; a view that is in line with the broad concept of health defined by the WHO (WHO, 1988).

3.2 The case of Andalusia

Today, all women in Andalusia have the right to request epidural analgesia during labour in the public hospitals of the region, irrespective of their size, type, or location.

The fact that epidural analgesia is now a reality is reflected in both the services portfolio of Andalusian hospitals and data gathered through annual surveys of user satisfaction with hospital care in Andalusia conducted by the Institute for Advanced Social Studies/Spanish National Research Council (IESA-CSIC).

As regards the services portfolio[2], Table 1 shows an increase in the total percentage of assisted births with epidural analgesia. The first year for which data are available is 2003, when epidural analgesia was used in one of every four deliveries at a public hospital in Andalusia. In 2009, this proportion rose to more than 1 in 2 deliveries.

Year	Mean in Andalusia
2003	25.4
2004	38.9
2005	47.1
2006	52.7
2007	53.1
2008	54.5
2009	56.3

Table 1. Percentage of assisted vaginal deliveries with epidural analgesia of all births in Andalusian hospitals

Data from surveys give very similar results, showing again that the use of epidural analgesia during labour is widespread among women giving birth in Andalusia. According to the responses given by the women themselves, the percentage of all births with epidural analgesia increased from 26% in 2000 to 64% in 2010. One reason for this widespread use is no doubt due to the fact that epidural analgesia is offered universally at all Andalusian hospitals. Women who underwent assisted deliveries in 2000 (14%) indicated that epidural analgesia was not available in the hospital where they gave birth; a percentage that decreased by around 6% mainly after 2004, and has maintained a downward trend to the present. In 2010, only 1.4% of women indicated that they were not allowed to use epidural analgesia because it was not available at the hospital where they gave birth (see Table 2).

In the first years that the study was conducted, important differences were found regarding the type of hospital. In general terms type A hospitals (regional hospitals) showed lower percentages of users who were not allowed to use epidural analgesia in the early years, while this occurred in type B hospitals (specialty) at first, and in type C and D hospitals (county I and county II hospitals) in following years. Since 2006, the gap between hospitals has narrowed, with all hospitals showing very low values that have practically equalled out.

[2] According to data on the percentage of assisted vaginal deliveries with epidural analgesia of all assisted deliveries by hospital based on hospital databases. The data were provided by the Andalusian Health Service and are available at: www.juntadeandalucia.es/servicioandaluzdesalud.

Year	Type A	Type B	Type C	Type D	Total
2000	9.1	18.7	14.9	13.7	13.5
2001	1.1	1.6	3.1	2.4	2.0
2002	8.0	6.2	13.4	9.2	9.1
2003	10.6	7.5	16.0	9.4	10.5
2004	3.7	3.4	11.1	6.1	5.9
2005	5.4	1.6	9.1	3.6	4.6
2006	2.7	1.8	5.2	2.8	3.1
2007	2.1	2.5	4.5	2.6	2.8
2008	3.3	1.2	3.2	2.6	2.6
2009	0.8	1.2	4.4	0.7	1.6
2010	1.7	0.4	2.5	1.3	1.4

Table 2. Response rate per year for the response category "*Did not use epidural analgesia because it was not allowed or it was not available at the hospital*"

4. Demand for epidural analgesia

But the use of epidural analgesia not only depends on the supply, that is, the fact that it is available and offered at hospitals. It also depends on women's own choice, who once informed can freely decide whether or not to make use of this pain relief method.

4.1 Characteristics of demand for obstetric epidural analgesia

Let us now analyse the characteristics of women requesting epidural analgesia during labour in Andalusian hospitals. If using or not using this type of anesthesia during labour is distributed randomly, we could only examine whether use has increased or decreased. However, as shown in an earlier study by our research group (Biedma -Velázquez et al., 2010), women who reject the use of epidurals have clearly defined characteristics, as we will discuss in the following pages.

The IESA-CSIC, in collaboration with the Andalusian Health Service (SAS), systematically conducts a survey of users of Andalusian hospitals to analyse their satisfaction with the services delivered. These surveys include a section dedicated to delivery care practices in which respondents are asked if they were administered an epidural. If they answer no, they must indicate the reason (e.g. did not consider it opportune, could not do so due to the characteristics of the birth that impeded using the epidural such as a cesarean section, the birth occurred very quickly and there was not enough time to administer it, complications, the service was not provided in the hospital, and others).

The percentage of women who choose epidural analgesia during labour is on the rise in Andalusia. This is due firstly to the increasing provision of this method at hospitals belonging to the Andalusian Public Health System (SSPA), and secondly to the increasing number of women who decide to use this method (see Table 3). Similarly, the percentage of women who state that they were unaware that they could request epidural analgesia during childbirth has also decreased.

Year	Yes	No, because I didn't consider it to be opportune	No, because I didn't know that I could request it	No, because it was not allowed/wasn't available at the hospital	No because I had a cesarean section/general anesthesia	No, because there was no time, it was very quick
2000	26.2	37.6	5.6	13.5	8.0	-
2001	36.7	52.4	6.6	2.0	0.0	-
2002	36.1	41.3	3.5	9.1	7.6	1.8
2003	45.0	35.6	1.9	10.5	6.9	0.0
2004	53.6	19.9	1.2	5.9	5.4	14.0
2005	58.4	17.9	0.9	4.6	4.6	13.7
2006	64.2	13.7	0.7	3.1	3.6	14.7
2007	60.8	16.2	0.7	2.8	4.6	14.8
2008	61.5	16.1	1.1	2.6	3.8	14.8
2009	66.4	12.8	0.4	1.6	5.1	13.7
2010	64.3	12.4	0.3	1.4	7.6	14.1

Table 3. Percentage of responses to the question "*Did you have epidural analgesia?*" by year

As shown in the table, the percentage of women who receive epidural analgesia during childbirth in Andalusian hospitals has increased by 250% since 2000, while the number of women who expressly reject this method of pain relief has dropped by an even higher percentage (3 times). In 2010 only 12% of the women surveyed rejected epidural analgesia as they did not consider it to be necessary or opportune.

However, although the number of women who decide not to use this type of anesthesia in a voluntary and conscious manner has decreased, they still account for a relatively significant portion of all women who give birth, particularly in a social context in which suffering pain is viewed as being pointless. Our objective is therefore to analyse whether these women have certain characteristics or whether the rejection of epidurals by mothers giving birth in public hospitals of Andalusia is randomly distributed.

To facilitate the analysis, and because certain answers do not depend on the express wishes of the expectant mother but on external circumstances (i.e. unavailability of epidural analgesia in the hospital or complications at birth), we consider only two possible answers: "Yes" and "No, because I did not consider it opportune" (see Figure 1). Not being aware of epidural analgesia was not taken into account either as only 0.3% of respondents gave this answer in 2010.

As shown in Figure 1, in 2000 a larger number of women rejected epidural analgesia than those who used it during childbirth, with a 17.8 point difference between rejection and use. The year 2002 marked a turning point in the use of epidurals as these two values showed similar percentages (53.4 and 46.6), with only a 6.7 point difference in favour of not using this pain relief method. This is the smallest difference observed across the time series between the two alternatives. From that year onwards, the difference continued to increase in a gradual but steady manner through 2010 when a difference of more than 67 points was observed between rejection and use (16.2 and 83.8).

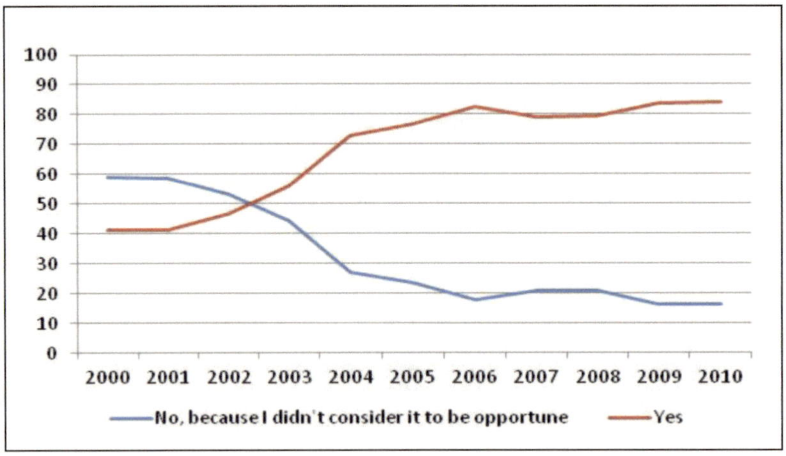

Fig. 1. Percentage of response to the question "Were you given an epidural during labour?" with only two response categories. Total years (2000-2010)

To analyse the characteristics of women who refuse epidural analgesia as opposed to those who choose to use it, we performed a cluster analysis in two phases using the SPSS 12.0 statistical package and subsequent versions. This method allows categorical and numeric variables to be entered jointly in order to group respondents according to common characteristics in different variables. After grouping the respondents, Pearson chi-square tests were performed to establish differences in the proportions between the clusters in the variables that formed them.

The results gave rise to three clusters. Specifically, women who gave birth in a hospital of Andalusia from 2000 to 2010 can be divided into 3 groups according to their sociodemographic characteristics (educational attainment, employment status and income) and use or not use of epidural analgesia. A total of 12,501 women were classified following this procedure. As shown in Figure 2, the 3 groups are comprised of different numbers of women.

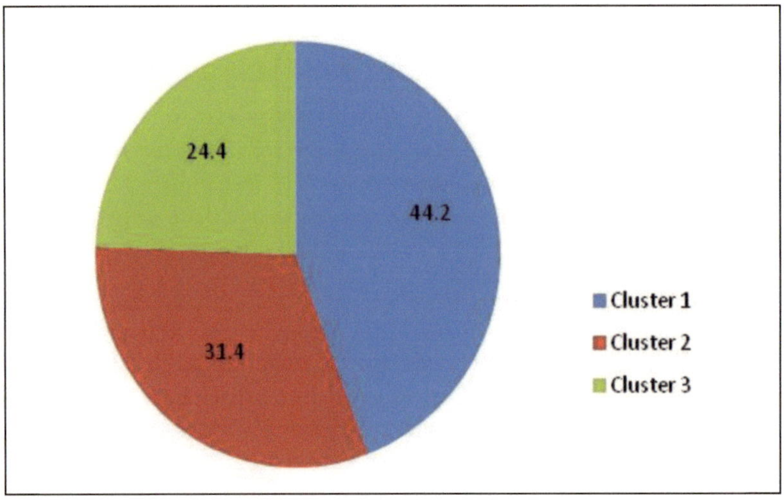

Fig. 2. Percentage of women in each cluster

We obtained three homogeneous groups taking into account the use of epidural analgesia during childbirth and the main sociodemographic characteristics of each such as educational attainment, income level and employment status.

Briefly, cluster 1 consists of women who behave close to the average values regarding their choice of epidural analgesia. These are women of all educational levels, employment status and income. As shown in Figure 3, cluster 1 contains women with differing levels of education, including a few with informal education. Regarding employment status, this group has the lowest number of employed women, with the majority belonging to another employment status (unemployed, students, etc.) or those who define themselves as housewives. Finally, family income (total income contributed by different members of the family) generally shows a similar distribution to that of the overall population. Cluster 1 is the largest group and comprises 44% of the women studied.

Cluster 2 is positioned well below the average with regard to the use of epidural analgesia during labour. The women in this cluster are mostly housewives, although there are some who work or have a different employment status. None of the women have a higher than primary school education. This is undoubtedly its main characteristic. In terms of the economic status of the family, cluster 2 mainly includes women from low-income families.

Finally, cluster 3 shows a higher than average use of epidural analgesia. It is interesting to note that all the women in this group work outside the home, have a secondary or university education and a higher family income than the women in the other two groups.

As can be observed, there are fundamental differences between clusters 2 and 3 in terms of both the use of epidural analgesia and the sociodemographic characteristics that define them.

The following graphs (see Figure 3) show the composition of each cluster according to their sociodemographic characteristics.

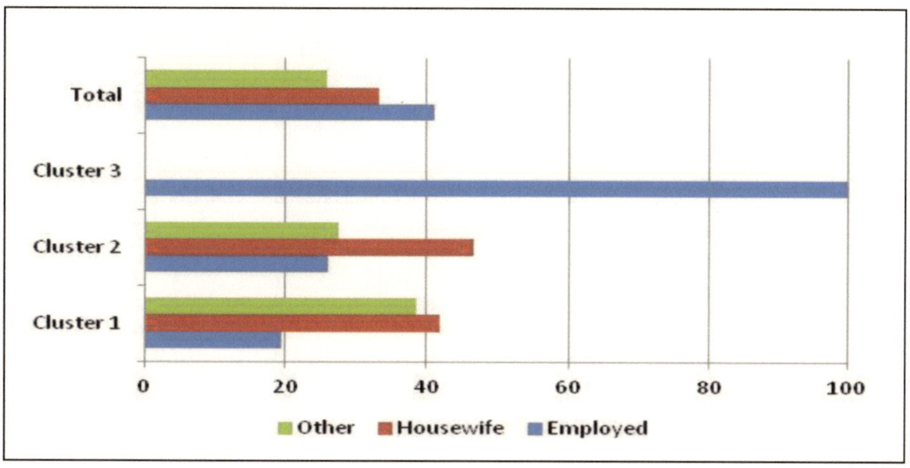

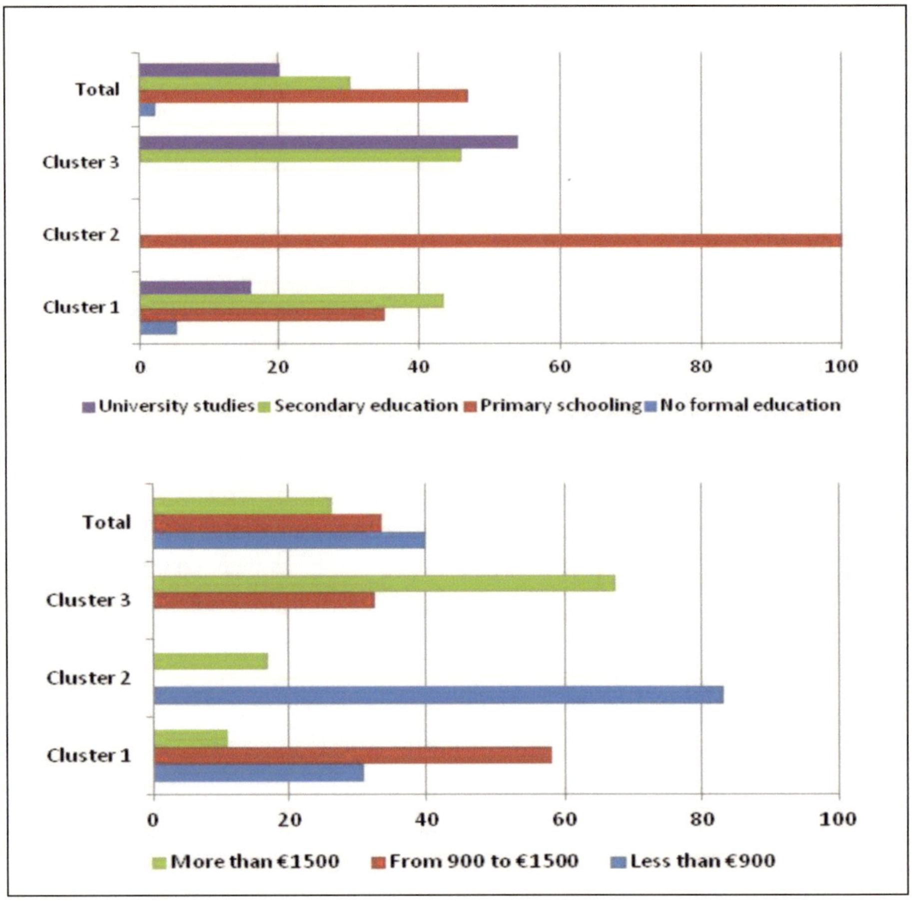

Fig. 3. Composition of the clusters according to employment status, educational level, and family income

Table 4 shows the differences between the three clusters regarding the use of epidural analgesia. Specifically, 39.1% of the women in cluster 2 indicated they did not use epidural analgesia during labour because they did not consider it opportune, while this percentage drops to 21.8% for cluster 3; a difference of more than 17 points. On the other hand, cluster 1 obtained a percentage that is close to the average for the rejection of epidural analgesia (32.1%).

		Cluster 1	Cluster 2	Cluster 3	Total
Epidural Analgesia	No, because I didn't consider it to be opportune	32.1%	39.1%	21.8%	31.8%
	Yes	67.9%	60.9%	78.2%	68.2%
Total		100%	100%	100%	100%
Sig 0.000					

Table 4. Percentage of response to the question *"Did you have epidural analgesia?"* in each cluster

In light of the data, it is interesting to note that the rate of voluntary refusal to have epidural analgesia during labour, and hence the acceptance of going through a painful experience when an alternative is available, differs among Andalusian women and is closely related to characteristics such as employment status, educational level and family income.

As shown in Table 3, the percentage of use of epidural analgesia during labour has increased significantly in Andalusia in recent years. However, there remains a group of women who explicitly reject the use of this method of pain relief, although they are clearly declining.

In short, the characteristics of women who refuse epidural analgesia in Andalusia differ from the characteristics of those who decide to use it (Biedma-Velázquez et al., 2010). This is highly relevant as it indicates that the social and cultural characteristics of women influence their decision to bear the pain of childbirth or not. The three groups have been defined according to income level, educational level and occupation and show different rates in terms of the use of epidural analgesia during childbirth in Andalusia. Family income was found to have a direct relationship to the use of epidurals; specifically women from higher income families are more likely to use this method of pain relief during childbirth. The same relationship was found for educational level, thus confirming that the lower the educational level, the higher the rejection of epidural analgesia and vice versa. Moreover, with regard to occupation, housewives are most likely to reject this pain relief method during childbirth, with clear differences observed between housewives and employed women and, to a lesser extent, between housewives and unemployed women or students.

When analysing educational level and occupation jointly (Figure 4), we see that the use of epidural analgesia increases among women with a higher educational level (values from 1 "not use" to 2 "use"). However, when analysing women according to their educational level, the lowest epidural usage rates occur among housewives for all the groups. Thus, although women with a university education use anesthesia during childbirth (always at a higher rate than women with no schooling), women with a university degree who most reject this pain relief method are housewives. Hence, being a housewife influences rejection of epidural analgesia, regardless of the mother's educational level.

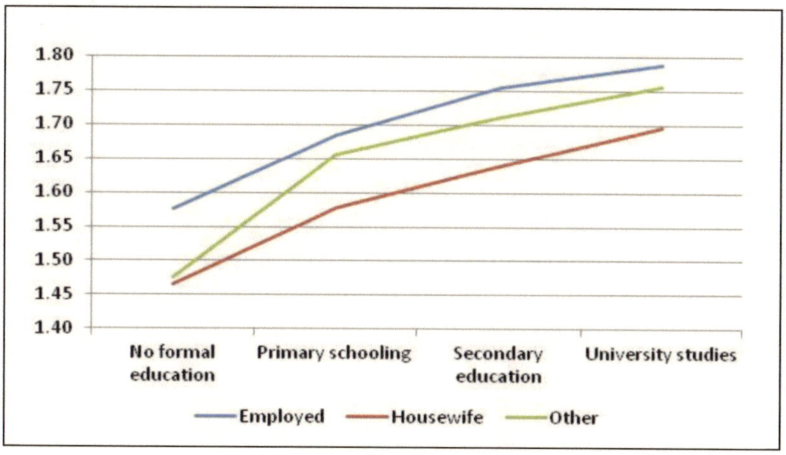

Fig. 4. Relationship between educational level and occupation in use of epidural analgesia during childbirth

The same is true when analysing family income and women's occupation. As can be seen in Figure 5, women with higher incomes show higher epidural usage rates, but being a housewife (regardless of economic status) has a negative impact on the use of this anaesthetic method, with significantly lower levels of use in all response categories.

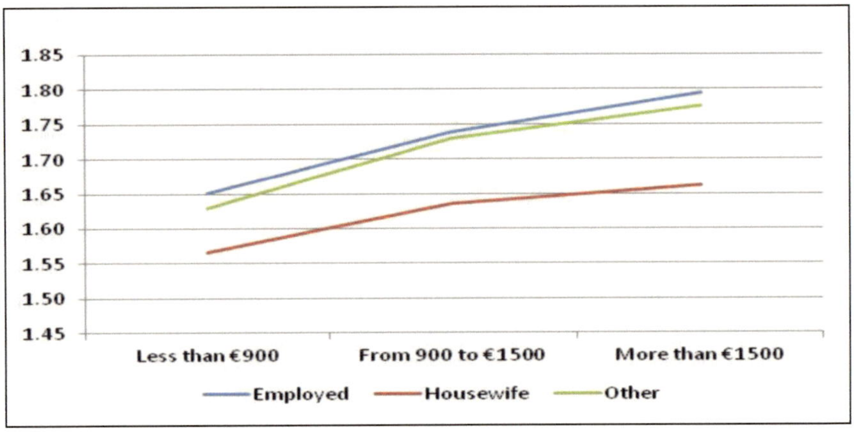

Fig. 5. Relationship between educational level and occupation in use of epidural analgesia during childbirth

In short, after performing a cluster analysis to determine the characteristics of women in the different groups that were formed according to sociodemographic variables and the variable "use or not use" anesthesia, we observe that the highest rejection rate occurs among women with low family incomes and a lower educational level; and as variables that impact on the rest, women who are housewives. As discussed in previous studies (Biedma-Velázquez et al., 2010), these characteristics define what we call "women folk" (Martín Criado, 2007a, 2007b). These women could be defined as being opposed to the new "modern" or "postmodern" lifestyles observed among women in Western societies. These women folk, although not in an excluding manner, could be defined by three areas of exclusion: labour, educational and economic. Hence their social integration implicitly involves assuming the role of social reproduction; a "traditional" lifestyle or role (Moreno, 2005) based on a socially acceptable discourse that advocates sacrifice and seeking the good of others before their own.

4.2 The "new culture" of natural childbirth

Despite the widespread use of epidural analgesia during childbirth, in recent years voices have been raised against administering this method of pain relief as well as the use of oxytocin. Some health professionals disagree about the benefits of this practice, warning of the risks of epidurals to both the mother and the foetus.

In addition, there is now a trend that could be called "post-modern", which extols the virtues of alternative birthing methods with minimal medical and biochemical intervention. The characteristics of the mothers who have taken up this trend differ greatly from those of "traditional" mothers in that women who choose alternative methods usually belong to a high socio-educational class and reject the use of epidurals for very different reasons based on highly elaborated biomedical arguments.

Today this new trend is known as "natural childbirth", although its meaning has yet to be conceptualised. Natural childbirth is grounded in the notion of an "ideal" delivery without monitoring or other instruments and with minimum medical and pharmacological intervention. However, the bases or method of this approach to childbirth have not been clearly established. Natural childbirth has emerged more as a movement against the medicalised model common in developed countries rather than as a specific practice on the grounds that practices removed from the "natural" are "unnatural". This practice, which is also known as "natural, non-medicalised childbirth", takes place under supervision and with minimal obstetric intervention only when strictly necessary to solve a problem. This method is in line with some of the recommendations made by the WHO in 1996 (Chalmers et al., 2001).

This movement emerged in England, the Netherlands and the Scandinavian countries driven by women's movements in the 1980s that put pressure on public institutions to allow women who felt that they had become a passive participant to take the reins of the birthing process.

The followers of this movement opt for home births attended by health professionals and with the necessary precautions in the event that they have to be transferred to a hospital. Some popular personalities who chose this method, such as Princess Marie Louise of Norway, were considered an example to follow. However, one should question if this system is actually viable if generalised, or whether these are practices that only a very small portion of the population with sufficient financial resources can afford and manage privately, at least in many countries. However, in countries like the Netherlands, where the cost of home births is covered by the public health system, over 30% of women give birth at home.

Furthermore, health professionals have yet to reach a consensus on the benefits of giving birth at home given that complications, which may initially appear to be minor, can lead to serious consequences if not handled quickly enough. Some maintain that it would be more feasible to try to recreate the home environment in the hospital.

Perhaps it would be wiser to advocate not using unnecessary medical interventions, rather than rejecting any type of medical intervention at all. In a like manner, the psychological and social as well as biological and physical aspects present during childbirth should be taken into account in order to attend to women in an integrated manner and ensure that labour and delivery are tailored to and meet the needs and preferences of women and their families. Indeed, this is the path that has already been taken by some health institutions (i.e. La Inmaculada Hospital in Almeria, Spain), which attempt to reduce the medicalisation of childbirth to a minimum, while monitoring the birth and permitting the mother and family to play a major role in the process.

5. Conclusion

As we have explained throughout this chapter, pain must be understood as a socially constructed concept involving psychological, educational, cultural, and sociological factors, which must be examined from the standpoint of subjective perceptions and context. Context influences the perception of pain, and how individuals address their suffering or the decision not to suffer. This issue was explored in section 4.1 of this chapter, where we discussed the socioeconomic factors that define Andalusian mothers who choose not to use epidural analgesia during childbirth.

Andalusian hospitals are making an effort to include epidural analgesia during labour in their clinical protocols by offering this method of pain relief where possible and when there is no risk to the baby or mother. In attempting to offer epidurals in a universal manner to all women who give birth, we must not overlook the fact that a portion of the demand side (in this case expectant mothers) hold a biased opinion about this method. This is a self-imposed bias, chosen in some way, but by no means lacking in social and political motives replete with elements of social inequality. Such biases respond to social and cultural stereotypes in which being a low-income woman with low educational level and a housewife are decisive factors in deciding to reject this healthcare service.

While other studies have reported similar differences with regard to the use of epidural analgesia discussed in this chapter (Fernández-Guisasola et al., 2004), they place greater emphasis on obstetric and biological variables, ignoring social and cultural aspects of the phenomenon. Without denying the effect and influence of the biological, psychological and obstetric (which were not analysed here due to the nature of our research) characteristics of the women studied, our work advocates the need to analyse this phenomenon from a social perspective. In line with Martín Criado (2007a, 2007b, 2004), we believe that women who reject the use of epidurals base their decision on values and beliefs supported in the traditional image of what it means to be a "good mother"; women who create their identity from the image that others have of them. It is an image that is characterised in part by women's complete devotion and capacity to sacrifice themselves for the good of others (in this case the baby before the mother) in the hope of earning social recognition in compensation for the sacrifices made (Tobias, 2002), or as a rite of passage and self-affirmation of a lived experience (Morris, 1991). In this sense, suffering becomes an exchange value (Matta, 2010) in which the baby in particular and the family in general acquire a "social debt" with the mother for her pain, based on the moral value that suffering should be rewarded.

A well-informed woman is fully aware of her right to refuse epidural analgesia during childbirth and demand that her decision be respected. Nonetheless, such rejection becomes a concern when it is the consequence of the social and gender inequality suffered by women who are not integrated in the labour market, have a low family income in which they do not participate directly, and have no formal education. Le Breton foresaw this trend when observing that the middle and upper classes reject pain as an enemy, while the lower, disadvantaged classes have a more submissive and resigned attitude towards pain and suffering (Le Breton, 1999). In a society like today's where, in general, avoidance of pain is highly valued over gratuitous or avoidable suffering, it is paradoxical and therefore worthy of explanation that a particular group of women choose to suffer when such suffering can be avoided (Illich, 1975; Levinas, 1993). Indeed, this could be another indicator of firmly-rooted gender behaviours and values that are characteristic of unequal patriarchal societies (Biedma-Velázquez et al., 2010).

In her anthropological studies, Margaret Mead (2001a, 2001b) discussed the effect of culture on pain during labour. She determined that if the expectant mother's culture views childbirth as a painful process, then most women in that society will have a painful childbirth. However, if giving birth is perceived of as a painless process, the experience is more likely to be painless (Macfarlane, 1977). In this case, education and culture are the main variables that condition the pain of childbirth. While pain cannot be perceived of as solely a cultural phenomenon, neither can pregnancy and childbirth be considered merely a biological event as they involve social and emotional aspects that influence the experience and the entire process; a process in which the mother cannot be relegated to a simply passive role (Castro & Bronfman, 1993).

Pain does not involve only the patient, or the expectant mother in this case, but their families and relations (Barragan-Solis, 2006; Kleinman, 1994), as well as the professionals that assist the patient and who give sense and meaning to the pain of others through compassion, acknowledgement and admiration; sentiments that the sufferer perceives and analyses as part of the meaning of such suffering, and which finally legitimises it or not, gives it meaning or not, and therefore makes it seem "useful" or not.

Today's hegemonic biomedical model offers multiple techniques, therapies and drugs to relieve pain, although not always with the desired results. However, relatively few works have examined the subjectivity let alone the "sociability" of pain. While it is accepted that pain may have a physical, emotional and psychological origin, regardless of its underlying causes, how pain is manifested will depend on the culture and society in which the individual has learned to perceive and interpret his or her pain. Despite this, little research has been conducted on the social context of those who suffer pain or the variables that may affect the interpretation, perception or even the intensity of pain. This lack of attention to the social responses of pain is undoubtedly due in part to the difficulties medical research encounters in analysing and empirically and "scientifically" testing such phenomena (Morris, 1991). It is difficult to analyse the social factors that influence the perception of pain; perceptions that vary from one society to another and from one moment in time to another because society is constantly changing. However, without such analyses our knowledge of pain will be incomplete when interpreting its meaning.

6. Acknowledgments

The authors would like to thank the Andalusian Health Service/Ministry of Health-Regional Government of Andalusia for their dedication and collaboration in the research project that has served as basis for this and many other works arising from the research group. We also acknowledge the valuable contributions, suggestions and support from our colleagues at the IESA-CSIC, especially Julia Ranchal and Sergio Galiano. In spite of these contributions, the authors assume full responsibility for the contents of this chapter. We do not want to finish without mentioning all the women who have selflessly contributed to this study through their responses. Without them this work would have been impossible.

7. Legislation

Decree 101/1995 of 18 April to determine the rights of parents and children during the birth process. BOJA 72 (17/05/1995).

Law 14/1986 of 25 April; General Law on Healthcare.

Law 41/2002 of 14 November regulating patient's autonomy and rights and obligations regarding information and clinical documentation. BOE 274 (15 November 2002).

Royal Decree 1030/2006 of 15 September establishing the common service portfolio of the National Health System and the procedure for updating the portfolio.

8. References

Barragán-Solís, A. (2006). El dolor crónico: una visión antropológica de acuerdo a familiares y pacientes [Chronic Pain: An Anthropologic View According to Relatives and Patients]. *Medicina Familiar*, Vol.8, No.2, pp.109-117, ISSN 1405-9657

Baszanger, I. (1992). Deciphering chronic pain. *Sociology of Health & Illness*, Vol.14, N°.2, pp.181-215, ISSN 0141-9889

Bayes, R. (1998). Psicología del sufrimiento y de la muerte. [Psychology of suffering and death]. *Anuario de Psicología* , Vol.29, No.4, pp.5-17, ISSN 00665126

Biedma-Velázquez, L.; García-de-Diego, JM. & Serrano-del-Rosal, R. (2010). Análisis de la no elección de la analgesia epidural durante el trabajo de parto en las mujeres andaluzas: "la buena sufridora". *Rev Soc Esp Dolor*, Vol.17, No.1, pp.3-15, ISSN 1134-8046

Bonica, JJ. (1990). *History of pain concepts and therapies. The management of pain.* 2nd edn. Lea & Febiger, Vol.1, ISBN 0812111222, Philadelphia

Breivik, H.; Collett, B.; Ventafridda, V.; Cohen, R. & Gallacher, D. (2006). Survey of chronic pain in Europe: Prevalence, impact on daily life, and treatment. *European Journal of Pain*, Vol.10, pp.287-333, ISSN 1090-3801

Calderón, E.; Martínez, E.; Román, MD; Pernia, A.; García-Hernández, R. & Torres, L (2006). Remifentalino intravenoso mediante infusor elastromerico frente a meperidia intramucular. Estudio comparado en analgesia obstetrica. *Rev Soc Esp Dolor*, Vol.13, N°7, pp.462-467, ISSN 1134-8046

Campuzano, C. (2007) Guidelines for obstetric epidural analgesia within a famework of innovatine managementand quallity and safety criteria [Protocolo de analgesia epidural obstétrica en el contexto de la gestión innovadora de la asistencia y de los citerios de calidad y seguridad] *Rev Soc Esp Dolor*, Vol.14, No.2, pp.117-124, ISSN 1134-8046

Chalmers, B.; Mangiaterra, V. & Porter, R. (2001). WHO principles of perinatal care: the essential antenatal, perinatal, and postpartum care course. *Birth*, Vol.28, N°.3, pp.202-207, ISSN 1523-536x

Castro, R. & Bronsfman, M. (1993). Teoría feminista y sociológia médica: bases para una discusión. *Cad Saúde Publ Río de Janeiro*, Vol.9, N°3, pp.375-394, ISSN 0102-311X

Cockerham, WC. (2002). *Sociología de la Medicina*. Pearson Education, ISBN 84-205-3084-0, Madrid

De la Torre, MR. & Pérez-Iraola, MP. (2002). Analgesia epidural del parto: ropivacaína vs bupivacina. *Rev Soc Esp Dolor*, Vol.9, pp.441-446, ISSN 1134-8046

Fernández, MA.; Ros, J. & Villalonga, A. (2000). Fallos en la analgesia epidural obstétrica y sus causas. *Rev. Esp. Anestesiol. Reanim*, Vol.47, pp.256-265, ISSN 0210-3591

Fernández-Guisasola, J. (2003). *Analgesia epidural obstétrica: organización y aspectos clínicos en un hospital general*. Unv. Compl Madrid, ISBN 84-669-2118-4, Madrid.

Fernández-Guisasola, J.; Rodriguez, G.; Serrano, ML.; Delgado, T.;García, S. & Gómez-Arnau, JI. (2004). Analgesia epidural obstétrica: relación con diversas variables obstétricas y con la evolución del parto. *Rev. Esp. Anestesiol. Reanim*, Vol.51, pp.121-127, ISSN 0210-3591

Franco, A. (1999). El dolor en la historia. *Rev Soc Esp Dolor,* Vol.6, pp.261-262, ISSN 1134-8046

Greenspan, JD.; Craft, RM.; LeResche, L.; Arendt-Nielsen, L.; Berkley, K.; Fillingim, RB.; Gold, MS.; Holdcroft, A.; Lautenbacher, S.; Mayer, A.; Mogil, J.; Murphy, AZ. & Traub, RJ. (2007). Stuydying sex and gender differences in pain and analgesia: A consensus report. *Pain,* Vol.132, Suppl.1, pp.26-45, ISSN 0304-3959

Guevara-López, U.; Córdova-Domínguez, JA.; Tamayo-Valenzuela, A.; Ramos, E. & Martínez-Espinoza, H. (2004). Desarrollo de los parámetros de práctica para el manejo del dolor agudo. *Revista Mexicana de Anestesiología,* Vol.24, No.4, pp.200-204, ISSN 0185-1012

Hanna, M.; Tuca, A. & Thipphawong, J. (2009). An open-label, 1-year extension study of the long-term safety and efficacy of one-daily OROS hydromorphone in patients with chronic cancer pain. *BMC Palliative Care,* Vol.8, No.14, pp.1-13, ISSN 1472-684X

Herrera, C. & Durán, MA. (1995). Las demandas de trabajo no monetarizado (DETRANME) de los ancianos. *Política y Sociedad,* Vol.19, pp.117-138, ISSN 1130-8001

Illich, I. (1975). *Némesis medica: la expropiación de la salud.* Barral editores, ISBN 84-7658, Barcelona

International Association for the Study of Pain [IASP] (1979). Pain terms: a list with definitions and notes on usage. *Pain,* Vol.6, pp.249-252, ISSN 0304-3959

Kirmayer, LJ. (2008). Culture and the metaphoric mediation of pain. *Transcult Psychiatry,* Vol.45, Nº2, pp.318-338, ISSN 1363-4615

Kleinman, A. (1994). *Pain and Resistance:The Delegitimation and Relegitimation of Local Worlds..* In Delvecchio, MJ.; Brodwin, PE.; Good, BJ. & Kleinman, A. *Pain as Human Experience. An Anthropological Perspective.* Chp.6, pp.169-197, University of Californa Press, ISBN 0-520-07512-9, Berkeley

Krivoy, S.; Tabasca, M.; Adelaide, W. & Díaz, M. (2010). *El dolor en la historia.* En Soulie, A. & Briceño-Iragorry, L. (ed.). Colección Razetti. Vol.X. Cap.6, Editorial Ateproca, pp.163-224, ISBN 978-980-6905-71-9, Caracas

Le Breton, D. (1999). *Antropología del dolor.* Ed. Seix Barral, ISBN 84-322-0833-7, Barcelona

Le Bretón, D. (2010). Pain and the care relationship. *Soins,* Vol.749, pp.34-5, ISSN 0253-0465

Leriche, R. (1937). *Cirugía del dolor.* Ed. Morata, ISBN 84-458-0374-3, Barcelona

Levinas, E. (1993). El sufrimiento inútil. En Levinas, E. *Entre nosotros. Ensayos para pensar en otro.* Pre-textos. ISBN 978-84-7213-138-5, Valencia

Loeser, JD. & Melzazck, R. (1999). Pain: an overview. *Lancet,* Vol.353, Nº9164, pp.1607-1609, ISSN 0140-6736

Macfarlane, A. (1977). *The psycholoy of childbirth.* Harvard University Press, ISBN 0-674-72106-3, USA

Martín-Criado, E. (2004). El valor de la buena madre. Oficio de ama de casa, alimentación y salud entre las mujeres de clases populares. *RES,* Vol.4, pp.93-118, ISSN 1578-2824

Martín-Criado, E. (2007a). El conocimiento nutricional apenas altera las prácticas de alimentación: el caso de las madres de clases populares en Andalucía. *Revista Española de Salud Pública,* Vol.81, pp.519-528, ISSN 2173-9110

Martín-Criado, E. (2007b). La dieta desesperada. Algunas consideraciones sociales que obstaculizan el control del peso entre madres de clases populares. *Trastornos de la Conducta Alimentaria,* Vol.6, pp.578-599, ISSN 1699-7611

Martins, RJ.; García, AR.; Garbin, CA. & Sundeleld, ML. (2008). The relation between socio-economic class and demographic factors in the ocurrence of temporomandibular joint dysfunction. *Cien Saude Colet*, Vol.13, Nº2, pp.2089-2096, ISSN 1413-8123

Matta, J. (2010). Cuerpo, sufrimiento y cultura; un análisis del concepto de „tecnicas corporales" para el estudio del intercambio lástima-limosna como hecho social total. *Cuerpos, Emociones y Sociedad*, Vol.2, pp.27-36, ISSN 1852-8759

Mead, M. (2001a). *Sex and temperament in three primitive societies*. Perenniol and Imprint of HarperCollins, ISBN 0-6093495-6, New York.

Mead, M. (2001b). *Coming of Age in Samoa: a psychological study of primitive youth of western civilisation*. Perenniol Classic, ISBN 0-688-05033-6, New York.

Mogil, J. (2004). *The Genetics of Pain*. IASP Press, ISBN 978-0-931092-51-0, Montreal

Moreno, A. (2005). Empleo de la mujer y familia en los regímenes de bienestar del sur de Europa en perspectiva comparada. Permanencia del modelo de varón sustentador. *RES*, Vol. 112, pp.131-163, ISSN 1578-2824

Morris, DB. (1991). *The culture of pain*. University of California Press, ISBN 0-520-08276-1 Berkeley, Los Angeles-Oxford

Moscoso, J. (2002). *Dolor privado, sensibilidad pública*. En Barona JL, Mocoso J, Pimentel J. *La ilustración de las ciencias. Para una historia de la objetividad.*. Biblioteca Valenciana, Cap. 6, pp.137-151, ISBN 84-370-5503-2, Valencia

Pagés, F. (1921). Anestesia metamérica. *Rev Esp Cir*, Vol.3, pp.121-148, ISSN 0009-739X

Pérez, J.; Abejón, D. & Ortiz, JR. (2005). El dolor y su tratamiento a través de la historia. *Rev Soc Esp Dolor*, Vol.12, pp.373-384, ISSN1134-8046

Pérez-Cajaraville, J.; Abejón, D.; Ortiz, JR. & Pérez, JR. (2005). El dolor y su tratamiento a través de la historia. *Rev Soc Esp Dolor*, Vol.12, pp.373-384, ISSN 1134-8046

Rohfs, I.; Borrel, C.; Anitua, C.; Artazcaz, L.; Colomer, C. & Escribá, V. (2000) La importancia de la perspectiva de género en las encuestas de salud. *Gac. Sanit.* Vol. 14, Nº2, pp.146-155, ISSN 0213-9111

Starfield, B. (2002). Equity and health: a perspective on nonrandom distribution of health in the population. *Pan. Am. J. Public. Health*, Vol.12, Nº6, pp.384-387, ISSN 1020-4989

Suvienen, TI.; Reade, P.; Kemppainen, P.; Könönen, M. & Dworkin, SF. (2005). Review of aetiological concepts of temporomandibular pain disorders: towards a biopsychosocial model for integration of physical disorder factors with psychological and psychosocial illness impact factors. *Eur J Pain*. Vol.9, Nº6, pp.613-633, ISSN 1090-3801

Tobío, C. (2002). Conciliación o contradicción: como hacen las madres trabajadoras. *RES*, Vol.97, pp.155-186, ISSN 1578-2824

Torres, A. (1999). Más sobre la anestesia epidural obstétrica. *Rev Soc Esp Dolor*, Vol.6, pp.403-405, ISSN 1134-8046

World Health Organization [WHO] (1952). *Constitution of the World Health Organization.* Handbook of basic documents (5ª ed.). pp. 3-20, Ginebra, Pelais des Nations

World Health Organization [WHO] (1988). *Distritct health system in action. 10 years after Alma-Alta experiences and future directions*, Neubrandenburg

7

Actualities and Perspectives in Continuous Epidural Analgesia During Childbirth in Romania

Virgil Dorca[1], Dan Mihu[2], Diana Feier[3], Adela Golea[4] and Simona Manole[3]
[1]ATI III Clinic of Obstetrics and Gynecology "Dominic Stanca", Faculty of Medicine.
[2]Clinic of Obstetrics and Gynecology "Dominic Stanca", Faculty of Medicine,
[3]Radiology and Medical Imaging Clinic, Faculty of Medicine,
[4]University Emergency County Hospital,
University of Medicine and Pharmacy, Cluj-Napoca,
Romania

"To the woman he said, I will make your pains in childbearing very severe; with painful labour you will give birth to children"
(Genesis 3, 16)

1. Introduction

Starting from this biblical precept, Christian religions used to regard pain occurring at childbirth as divine punishment. Given the fact that childbirth pain is perceived as very severe and evaluated as more intense than toothache, phantom limb pain or even the ache caused by a fracture, with the progress of society, human condition and the status of women, childbirth pain has become ever more difficult to accept.

The epidural therapeutic administration of drugs was practically initiated in 1884, when Corning, a New York neurologist, administered cocaine through a needle inserted at level T11-T12 [Bonica J, Mc Donald JS, 1995]. It was not until 1901 that Cathelin [Cathelin MF, 1901] reported in France a caudal epidural anesthesia. In 1921, Pages used lumbar epidural anesthesia, and in 1931, Dogliotti described the method of locating the epidural space through "the technique of loss of resistance" (LOR) [Dogliotti AM, 1934; Abboud T et al., 1980]. The first use of lumbar epidural analgesia in obstetrics remains somewhat uncertain. In 1935, Graffagnino and Seyler [Bonica J, Mc Donald JS, 1995; Graffagnino P, Seyler LW, 1938] published in American literature the first reports on the use of epidural analgesia in obstetrics. In January 1947, Manuel Curbelo in Cuba used an ureteral catheter [Dogliotti AM, 1934; Graffagnino P, Seyler LW, 1938] inserted through a Tuohy needle and thus achieved the continuous epidural. Immediately after, Umstead and Dufresne applied this technique in obstetrics. In 1949, Cleland described the double catheter technique. In the 1950s, Bonica and Bromage described the superiority of lumbar epidural analgesia compared to caudal analgesia.

2. The situation of epidural analgesia in childbirth in Romania

Although epidural analgesia is becoming increasingly popular throughout the world, its applicability in Romania is still limited. In our studies, we have attempted to analyse the reasons for which women request or refuse epidural analgesia at childbirth, the level of knowledge of the participants in the study with regard to this method and the situation of epidural analgesia at childbirth in the main county hospitals, university clinics and private hospitals across Romania.

Starting from the premise that "maternal wish is a sufficient justification for alleviating pain during labour", as mentioned by the American College of Obstetrics and Gynaecology and the American Society of Anaesthesiologists [American Society of Anesthesiologists Task Force on Obstetric Anesthesia, 2007], it is important to understand the pain that occurs during labour. Epidural analgesia is a means of alleviating pain which is preferred by women in developed countries [Robert R, Gaiser RR, 2005]. In a study conducted by Minhas *et al.* (2005) [Minhas MR et al., 2005], 76% of the women knew that epidural analgesia was a method of alleviating pain; nevertheless, only 19% made use of this technique. From this point of view, we have attempted to conduct a "market study" regarding the situation of epidural analgesia in childbirth in Romania.

In our study, we have interviewed 205 parturients, evaluated by means of a questionnaire containing 12 sections, the collected data being compiled using Med Calc version 9.1.

Since the variables tested have not brought forth a normal distribution, the Kruskal-Wallis, Mann-Whitney tests and Spearman's correlation coefficient have been chosen as test patterns. With descriptive statistics (average, standard deviation, frequency tables), the *t test* has been utilised in comparing nominal data, while the chi-square test has been made use of for qualitative data. A confidence interval of 95% and $p < 0.05$ have been used in the evaluation.

In our study, 25,36 % of the parturients opted for epidural analgesia, namely a percentage of 84,61 of the parturients that were aware of the indications, advantages and potential disadvantages of the procedure (See Table 1).

A percentage of 86,27 of the women that did not give birth with epidural analgesia did not hold any information concerning the procedure. A painless labour had a positive effect on the parturients, due to an increase in maternal satisfaction, while providing them with the possibility to participate actively in the act of childbirth. The reasons why they chose to give birth with epidural analgesia was the fear of pain, or previous positive experiences, both personal and those of acquaintances. (See Table 2)

A high percentage of the parturients feared pain during labour (57,7%). In this study, the reasons for which they refused undergoing labour on epidural analgesia were the wish to have a natural childbirth, previous negative experience regarding epidural analgesia, negative experiences of other patients and fear of side effects. (See Table 3)

As shown by Bussche *et al.* [Bussche EV et al., 2007], the main factor that determined the parturients' decision was social influence. There are studies which report numerous factors that influence the decision to use epidural analgesia, such as age, level of education and health insurance status [Atherton MJ et al., 2004; Obst TE et al., 2001; Rust G et al., 2004; Salim R et al., 2005].

	Childbirth with epidural analgesia (n = 52)		**Childbirth without epidural analgesia (n = 153)**		
Characteristics	**N**	%	n	%	*p*
Age, years					
≤20	7	13,46	45	29,41	0,80
21-30	38	73,08	75	49,02	
≥30	7	13,46	33	21,57	
Level of education promoted					
Secondary School	2	3,85	53	34,64	**0,05**
High School	18	34,62	85	55,55	
University	32	61,53	15	9,81	
Knowledge regarding epidural analgesia in childbirth					
Yes	44	84,61	21	13,73	**0,02**
No	8	15,39	132	86,27	

Table 1. Characteristics of patients included in the study (N = 205)

Reasons	n	%
Fear of pain	30	57,70
Previous negative personal experience	12	23,07
Positive experience of other people	10	19,23

Table 2. Reasons why the parturients chose epidural analgesia (n = 52)

Reason	n	%
The wish to have a natural childbirth	7	33,40
Personal negative experience	5	23,80
Negative experience of other people	5	23,80
Fear of side effects	4	19,04
Advice of gynaecologist	6	28,57

Table 3. Reasons why the parturients refused epidural analgesia (n = 21)

A low percentage of epidural analgesia procedures during labour is noticed (25,36%), with a majority of 61,53% among patients that graduated from higher education. Most had been informed about these techniques of alleviating pain (84.61%). There was a significant difference with respect to the level of education between the group that benefited from epidural analgesia and the one that did not experience the procedure (p = 0,05). The women that gave birth without analgesia (74,64%) were mostly high school graduates (5,55%) and did not have sufficient information on epidural analgesia in childbirth (87,27%).

The argument that upholds this conclusion may be the fact that epidural analgesia is not largely utilised in childbirth in Romania. According to the 2009 statistics, epidural analgesia is used by approximately 78% of women in natural childbirths within private clinics. Even though the number of private clinics is not considerable in our country, they are more prone to promoting analgesia during labour, with a significant difference ($p<0,0001$) compared to university hospitals and county units. (SeeFig.1)

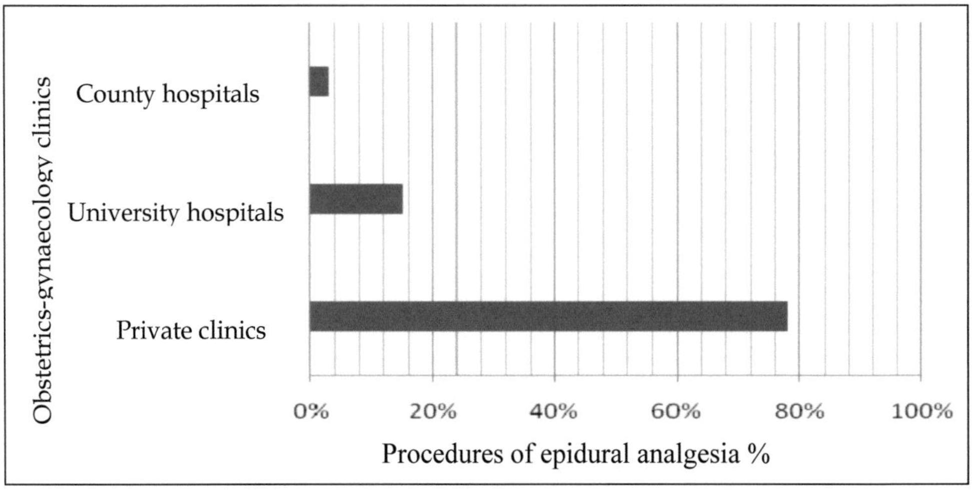

Fig. 1. The percentage of epidural analgesia procedures in the main obstetrics clinics in Romania

The very small percentage (3%) of the number of epidural analgesia in county hospitals may be explained by the staff's lack of experience and the shortage of appropriate materials [El-Hamamy E, Arulkumaran S, 2005]. Moreover, young doctors do not benefit from the proper environment so as to learn the correct procedure. Their internship in an obstetrics-gynaecology hospital is far too short to provide them with suitable experience. For this reason, there is a phenomenon of parturient migration from city and county hospitals to university and private ones. Parturients prefer hospitals with high-tech equipment and personnel with appropriate experience. A worrying aspect is the fact that the Romanian public does not have sufficient information on this topic and, moreover, public insurance programmes do not cover epidural analgesia at childbirth. Of the total number of women having undergone the procedure, only 4 (7,69%) experienced pain in the place of anesthesia. After childbirth, the latter stated they were displeased with epidural analgesia and that they would not encourage the use of this means of alleviating pain. The patients that benefited from epidural analgesia in childbirth without the side effects of the procedure exhibited a high level of satisfaction. El-Hamamy & Arulkumaran have shown that in this case, women did not feel pain during labour, childbirths occurred successfully and women were aware of all events during labour, while feeling comfortable [El-Hamamy E, Arulkumaran S, 2005].

It is our view that pregnant women have to be informed, by means of educational materials, in order to become aware of the directions, benefits, side effects and potential complications of this procedure. It is necessary to have qualified personnel in order to achieve a safe and painless childbirth for anyone who opts for pain alleviation during this event, through epidural analgesia [Dorca V et al., 2011].

3. PCEA vs CEI

In Romania, the question that arises regarding the administration of local anaesthetic refers to either "top-up" or CEI, although the unwanted side effects like intense motor block [Ferrante F M et al., 1994] are well-known, despite testing various dosages and combinations of anaesthetics [Ferrante F M et al., 1994; Van der Vyver M et al., 2002].

In our studies, we have used a method that is popular with developed countries and not in Romania, introduced in 1988 by D. Gambling (PCEA), in an attempt to reduce the side effects of the other methods, by looking for the drug, dosage and protocol that are ideal in the improvement of the childbirth process, while providing the parturient with psychological and physical comfort and increased maternal satisfaction [Ferrante F M et al, 1994; Van der Vyver M et al, 2002; Ferrante F M et al, 1991; Dorca V et al, 2009]. We have compared this method to one that is popular in Romania and used in the West since the 1980's, CEI [Gambling D R et al., 1988].

A number of 94 patients entered the study, as they were followed within the "Dominic Stanca" Clinic of Obstetrics and Gynaecology in Cluj-Napoca, so as to conduct an operational, prospective and randomised study.

The parturients were prospectively randomised in order to benefit from a continuous epidural infusion using levobupivacaine or patient-controlled epidural analgesia (PCEA), using the same substance. The patients that were eligible for the study were above the age of 18, ASA I, primipara/secundipara, they had asked epidural analgesia during labour upon admission, having a gestation time of over 37 weeks and exhibiting cranial presentation of the foetus. The minimum cervical dilatation at the moment of initialising epidural analgesia was of 3-4 cm, with uterine contractions at regular intervals of 5-6 minutes. General contraindications of epidural analgesia were the exclusion criteria from the study protocol. Cervical dilatation of over 6 cm was also among the exclusion criteria.

The protocol was conducted in the delivery room, with the patient sitting. At the L3-L4 level, a 20 G multi-orifice catheter was inserted with a Tuohy 18G B-Braun needle, using the LORS technique [Gadalla F et al., 2003]. The catheter was secured and its position verified with a 3 ml test dose of levobupivacaine 0,250 mg%. The patients that were selected for PCEA had the device installed and were instructed as to its functionality. The explanations focused on the manner in which they have to press the button that triggers the bolus dose and on the timing, which should coincide with the apparition of pain. It was expected that improvement should occur within a few minutes. Levobupivacaine 0,250 mg% 10 ml bolus was administered, followed by bolus upon request at 5 ml 0,125 mg%, with a *lock-out* period of 15 minutes and a total hourly dose of 20 ml. The patients that were administered a continuous epidural infusion were given the same bolus dose of 10 ml levobupivacaine 0,250 mg%, followed by a continuous infusion of levobupivacaine 0,125 mg%, 7 ml/hour, the total dose varying according to the duration of childbirth.

During labour, the foetus' heartbeats and uterine activity were monitored with the help of a cardiotocograph, along with the mother's blood pressure, respiratory frequency and haemoglobin oxygen saturation. The quantification of pain, using the visual analogical scale (VAS) [Paech M, 2000], which varies from 0 (painless) to 10 (most acute pain), was conducted prior to adding the catheter and, subsequently, every 15 minutes, until the time of expulsion.

The caudal development of the sensitive block grew with the gradual loss of cold sensation [Bromage P R et al., 1964]. The degree of the motor block was appreciated using the Bromage score (0 = no motor block: complete flexion of the knee and calf; 1 = impossibility to lift the leg in extension, knee movements; 2 = impossibility to flex the knee, calf movements; 3 = no calf or knee movements [Bromage P R et al., 1964]). For each patient, we followed the total dose of levobupivacaine utilised, the ratio demand/offer, the time necessary for dilatation, VAS evolution compared to dilatation, the level of maternal satisfaction, the foetus' state at birth (assessed by the neonatologist through the Apgar score, 1 and 5 minutes after birth), the manner of deliverance - vaginally, by caesarean or vacuum extraction. The need for supplementary involvement of medical personnel during labour was equally assessed. Maternal satisfaction was estimated subjectively by the mother according to the level of pain alleviation, the apparition of side effects such as nausea, vomiting, itching, backaches, dural post-puncture headache, both during analgesia and 24 hours after childbirth.

We have chosen for this study isomer L of bupivacaine in a concentration of 0,125 - 0,250 %, due to its low toxicity compared to racemic mixture and we have not used opioids or other adjuvants. Even though these concentrations are considered to be "high" [Owen MD et al., 1998; Meister GC et al., 2000] in studies that have used more diluted solutions with fentanyl as an adjuvant, no statistically significant differences were noticed with regard to the dose of local anaesthetic utilised, the quality of analgesia or maternal satisfaction, when they were compared to the results obtained when using "increased" concentrations [Meister GC et al., 2000; Lyons Gr et al., 2007].

The demographic, anthropometrical and obstetrical parameters of the patients included in the study show statistically significant differences with regard to motor block and instrumental childbirth (See Tables 4, 5).

Demographic and anthropometric parameters	CEI lot (53; 56,39%)	PCEA lot (41; 43,61%)	p*
Age (years)	27,02±1,23	26,20±1,92	0,1
Height (cm)	162,2 ±3,27	165,5±2,29	0,6
Weight (kg)	76,8 ± 8,5	78,5 ±9,2	0,4
Unipara patients	27 (50,94%)	25 (60,97%)	0,5

Data is expressed as average ± SD or number (%). SD=standard deviation.

Table 4. Demographic and anthropometric parameters of the patients included in the study

The results we have obtained reflect a significant difference from a statistical point of view with regard to the number of instrumental childbirths. 2 (4,86%) of the parturients from the PCEA lot required the obstetrician's instrumental intervention by vacuum extraction, a difference which is significantly lower compared to the CEI lot, 14 (26,41%), p<0,0001. This can be due to the intense motor block caused by continuous epidural infusion, which prevents the patient from collaborating during labour. The motor block with a Bromage score of above 2 does not enable the patient to use her abdominal muscles in order to facilitate the descent and positioning of the foetus' head. The patient group that benefitted from CEI presented a Bromage score between 2 and 3, which explains the large number of instrumental childbirths. (See Figure 2)

Obstetrical parameters	**CEI lot (53; 56,39%)**	**PCEA lot (41; 43,61%)**	**p***
Cervical dilatation (cm)	3,4 ± 1,1	3,1 ± 0,8	0,2
Duration of labour (minutes)	168,5 ± 123,1	188,3 ± 133,16	0,2
Total drug dose (ml)	39,4 (9,3-40,1)	35,3 (20–190)	0,08
Ratio demand/offer	0	1/1	NS
Sensitive block (VAS linearity)	T10-L3-L4	T10-L3-L4	NS
Motor block	21 (39,7%)	2 (4,87%)	**0,001**
Maternal satisfaction degree	High	High	
State of foetus (APGAR 5')	8,3 (8,12-10,20)	8,4 (8,23-11,02)	NS
Instrumental childbirth (vacuum extraction)	14 (5,66%)	2 (4,86%)	**<0,0001**
Childbirth by caesarean	8 (15,09%)	4 (9,75%)	0,09

Data is expressed as average ± SD, average (CI) or number (%). CI = confidence interval

Table 5. Obstetrical parameters of the patients included in the study

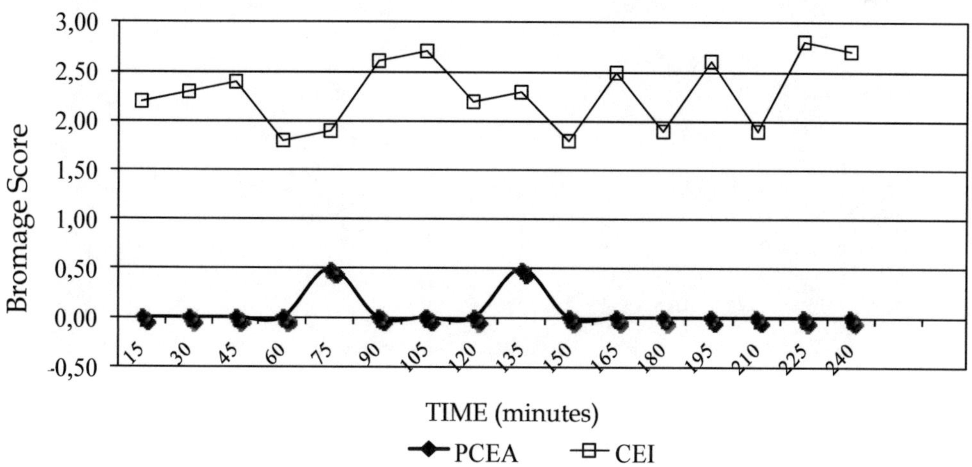

Fig. 2. Bromage score combined with the comparative time between the two lots (p<0,0001)

The patients from the PCEA lot maintain the linearity of the Bromage score below value 1, the low percentage of childbirths by vacuum extraction (4,86%) being one of the major advantages of this technique.

The motor block more frequently encountered in the CEI lot was significantly amplified on the right side. Speciality literature attempts to explain this by emphasising the exact spot of the dural puncture with the help of ultrasonography [Schlotterbeck H. et al., 2008], as we did in the case of 15 patients in collaboration with the Imaging Chair of the University of Medicine and Pharmacy in Cluj-Napoca. We thus managed to accurately determine bone markings, the distance between the skin and the epidural space, the position of the needle in the yellow ligament, the size of the epidural space and the presence/position of the catheter in the epidural space. (See Figures 3, 4, 5, 6)

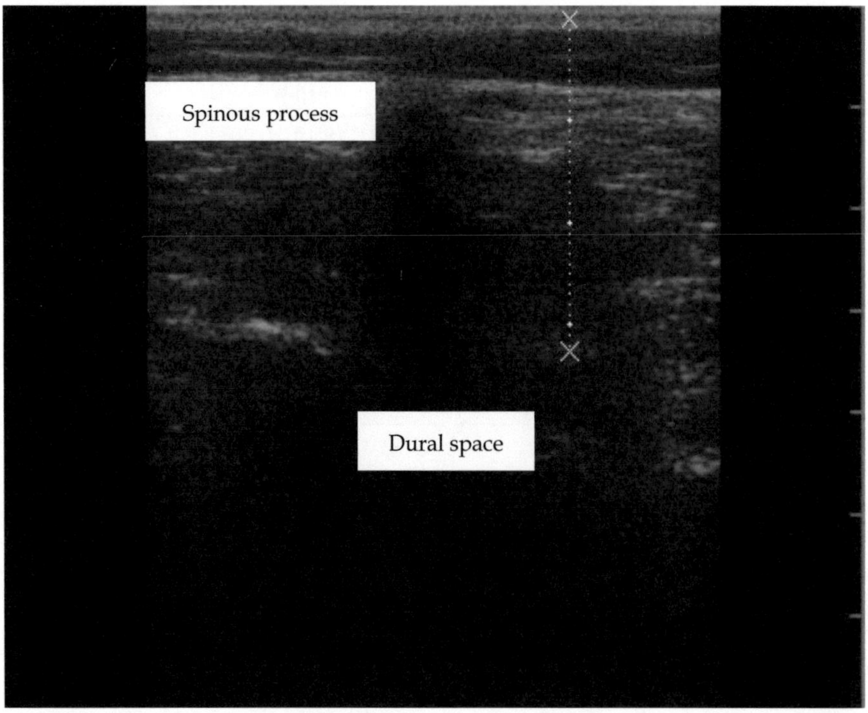

Fig. 3. Transversal section: the spinous process situated in the centre; the dural sac and distance evaluation at the tegument level

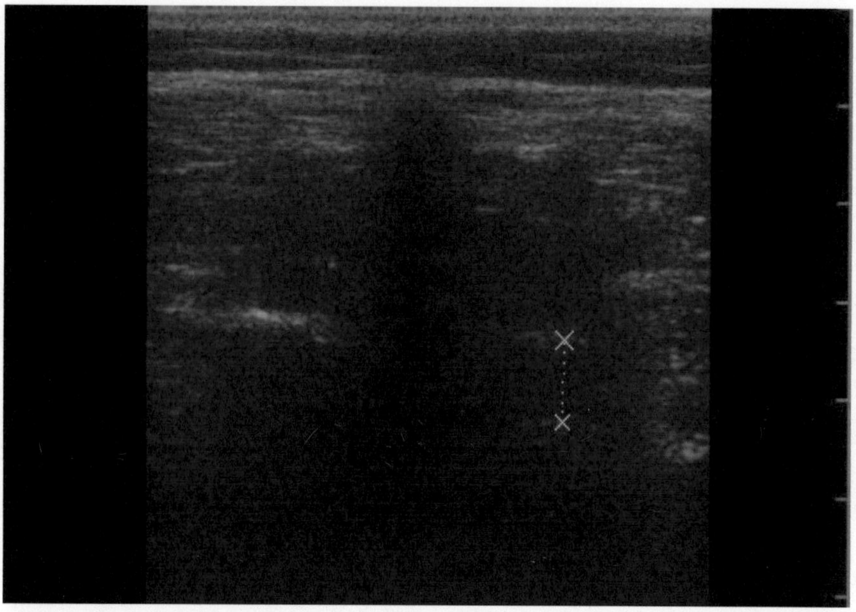

Fig. 4. Transversal section: the spinous process situated in the centre; measurement of the anteroposterior distance of the dural sac; view of the ligament and the posterior dura mater; vertebral body with posterior acoustic shadow

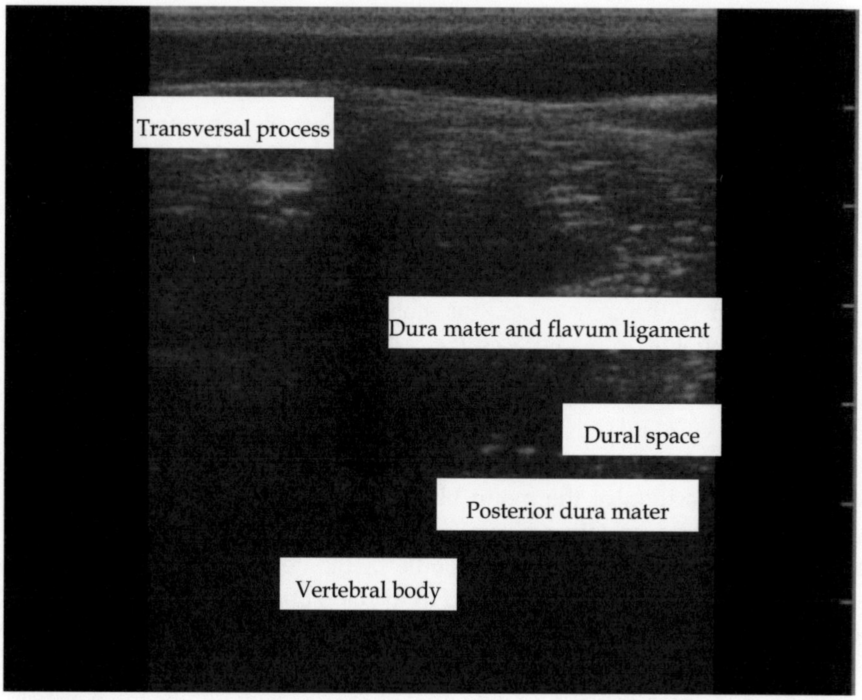

Fig. 5. Parasagittal section with the transverse apophysis (posterior shadow cone) and view of the dural space

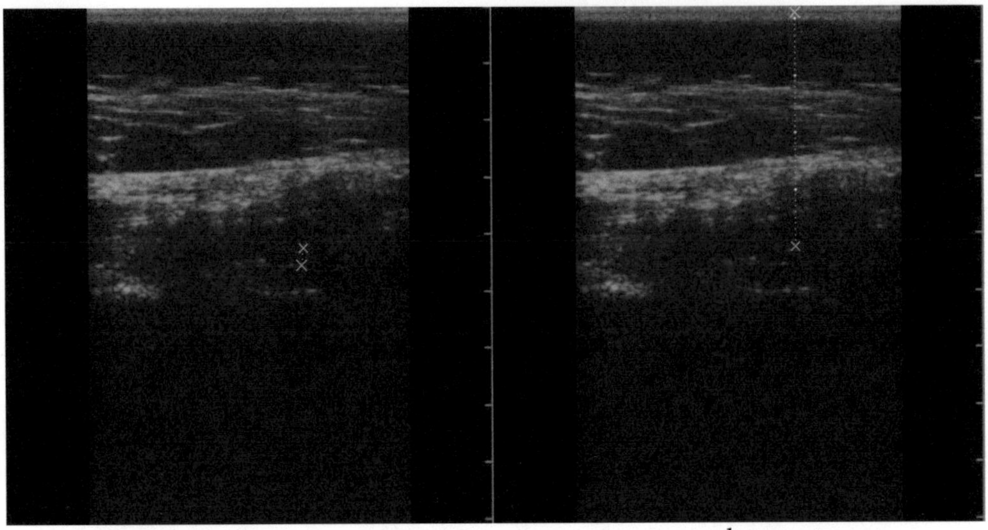

a. b.

Fig. 6. Parasagittal left section: a - view of catheter situated centrally in the dural sac;
b - measurement of the distance between the tegument and the position of the catheter

Despite the ecographic guidance, we have never managed to place the needle on the median line. (See Figure 7)

One explanation may be the dose and bolus concentration utilised (0,250mg% levobupivacaine), but due to the fact that subsequently, the concentration decreases and remains the same throughout labour, this is not justified. Attempting to explain the motor block, usually occurring asymmetrically (on the right), we photographed the catheters after their retreat from the epidural space. (See Photo 1)

Thus, one can notice the clear connection between the right side position of the catheter and the asymmetric motor block. In patients that did not experience any motor block, it can be noticed the median position of the catheter (See Photo 2), so the connection described between the position of the catheter and the motor block does exist. We have not managed to uncover the reason why in many cases, the catheter is situated laterally (especially on the right).

The PCEA lot receives 20 ml/hour of levobupivacaine 0,125mg% and does not develop any motor block, unlike the CEI lot, which is given a lower, but continuous dose, of 7 ml/hour. This favours the apparition of the motor block, probably due to the long period of time during which the substance "lingers" amongst nerve fibres at the level of the top of the catheter, managing in time to reach the middle of the nerve bunch at fibre Aα, which it blocks. (Figure 8). This lingering is favoured in the case of continuous infusion (7 ml/hour) and the fact that during one minute, just two drops are delivered, the anaesthetic substance not being able to diffuse on a long distance. We have also found that, in the case of a continuous infusion, there appears a single drop at the distal end of the three-orifice catheter (See Photo 3), whilst by administering the substance in bolus, it springs from all the three orifices (See Photo 4), its distribution being much more uniform and distant.

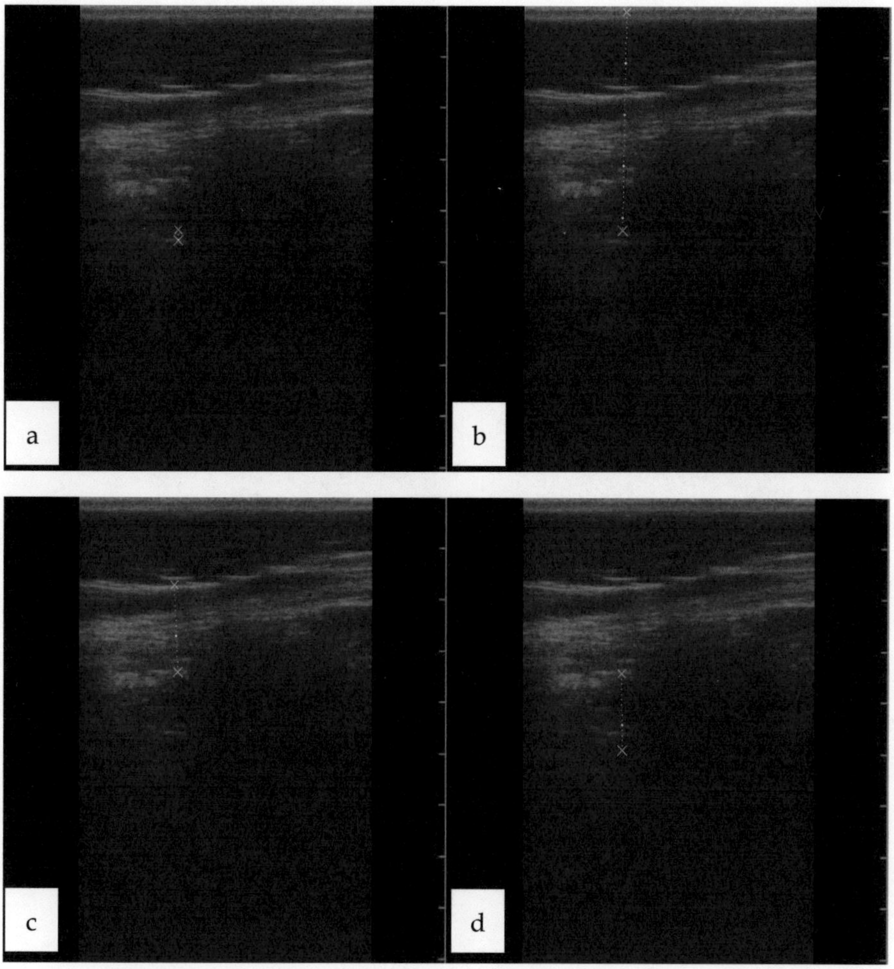

Fig. 7. Parasagittal left section: a - view of the catheter; b - measurement of the distance between the tegument and the position of the catheter; c- thickness of dura mater - flavum ligament; d- latero-lateral dimension of the dural sac, with a view of the right side of the catheter

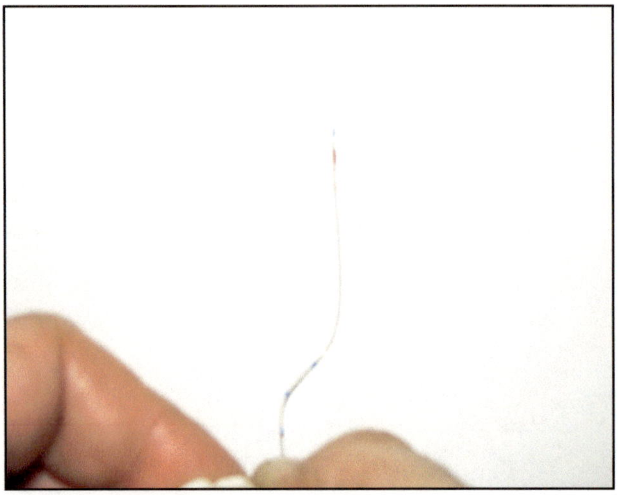

Photo 1. Position of the catheter on the right, after extraction from the epidural space

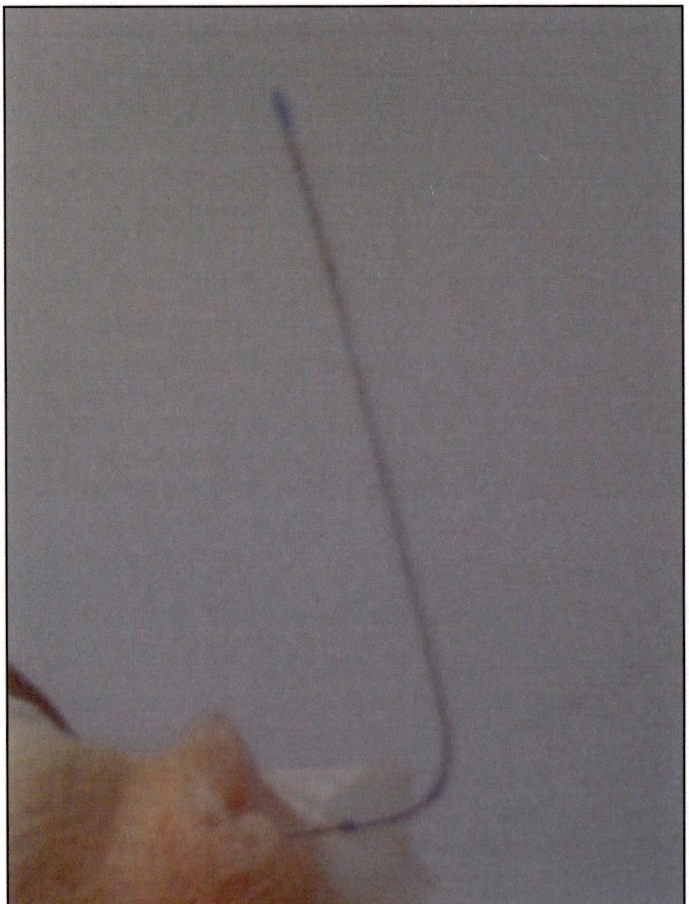

Photo 2. Median position of the catheter after extraction from the epidural space

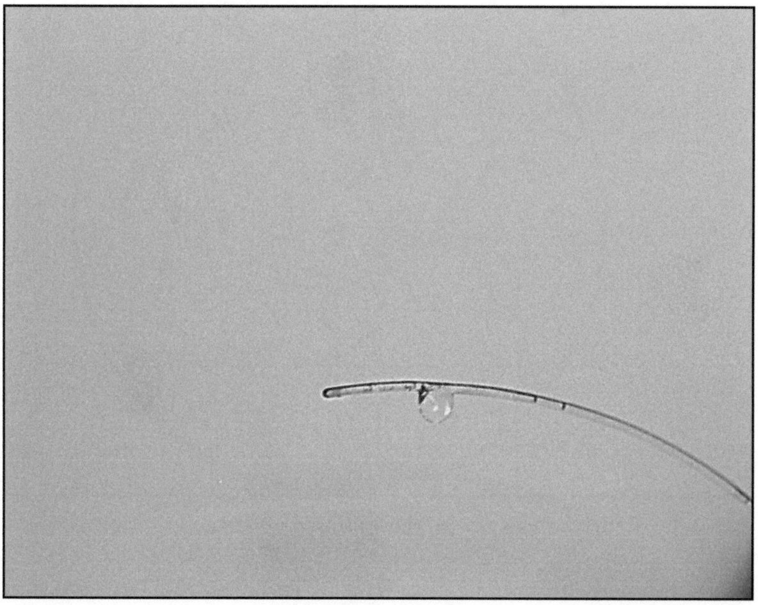

Photo 3. Illustrative image of the apparition of a single drop at the distal end of the catheter, following the administration of the analgesic substance in a continuous infusion

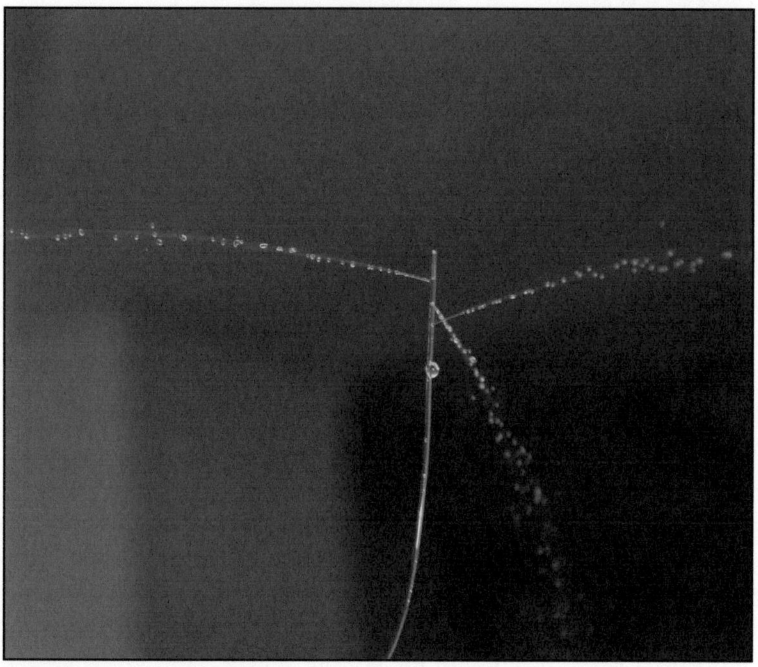

Photo 4. Administration of the analgesic substance in bolus

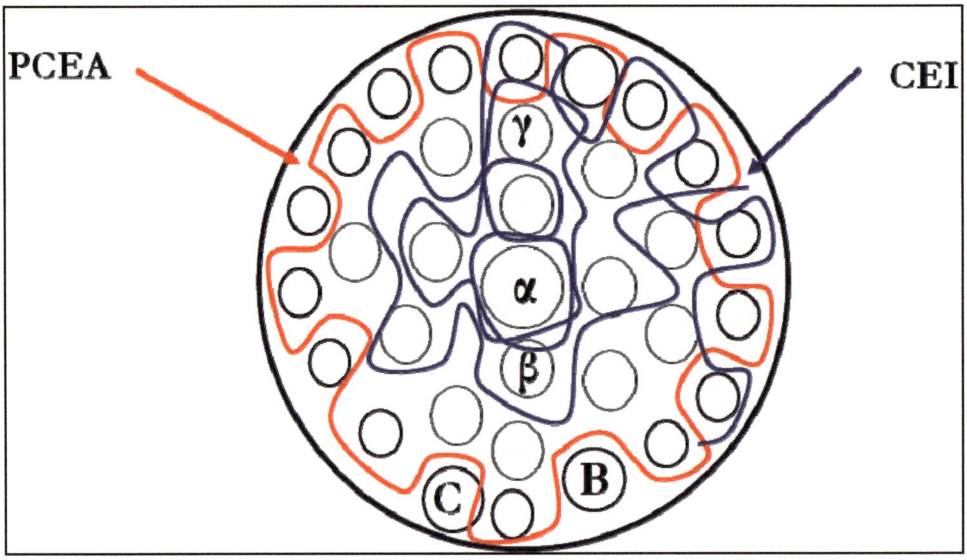

Represents the analgesic substance penetrating the periphery of the nerve fibre, using the PCEA method.

Represents the analgesic substance penetrating the periphery of the nerve fibre, using the CEI method.

Fig. 8. Schematic structure of the nerve fibre

Studies using MRI [Davidson EM et al., 2009], CT (See Figure 9), epiduroscopy, marked radioactive isotopes [De Biasi P et al., 2003] and studies on cadavers have demonstrated the existence of a vertical conjunctive septum and of horizontal septa which practically divide the epidural space [Aggarwal A et al., 2009]. These septa prevent the substance from diffusing amongst them, probably determining the asymmetry of the block. The small quantity of the substance infused using the CEI method may not succeed in distributing evenly throughout the epidural space. Even though the anterior epidural space is not well represented, in collaboration with our colleagues from the Chair of Imaging from the University of Medicine and Pharmacy in Cluj-Napoca, we have managed to emphasise the existence on this space, as well as of a median septum. (See Figure 10 a,b). Frequent boluses in PCEA enable the substance to diffuse more easily amongst these septa, which upholds the theory stating that this technique is a major determinant in the apparition, intensity and symmetry of the block. There are studies in the speciality literature that mention the fact that the behaviour of the anaesthetic substance according to density also contributes to the apparition of the motor block [Aggarwal A et al., 2009].

Hence, the isobaric substance remains in the proximity of the place of injection, the hypobaric substance ascends from the place of injection, while the hyperbaric one descends. Moreover, the density of the anaesthetic substance varies inversely proportional to temperature. According to these principles, an isobaric substance at room temperature will become isobaric at bodily temperature, and if the patient is in left lateral decumbency, the most frequently encountered position in the current practice, the substance will ascend on the right side, determining an asymmetrical motor block.

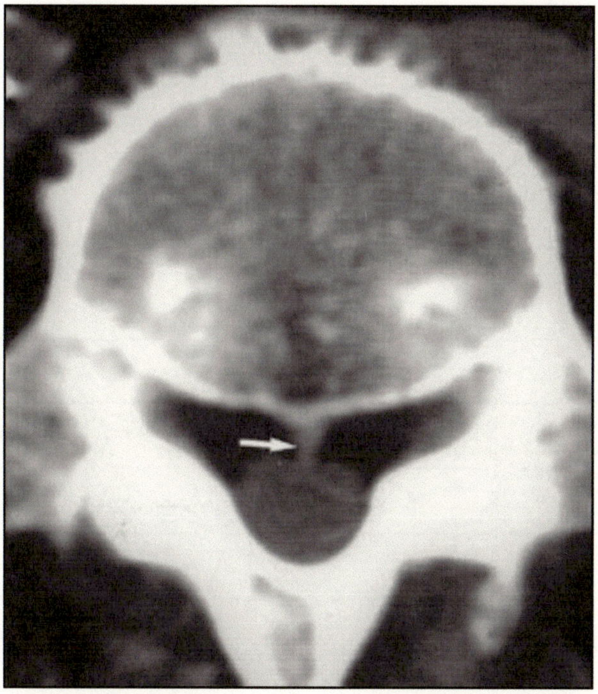

Fig. 9. CT axial section through vertebra S1. The median septum is clearly visible (arrow), dividing the epidural space into two separate compartments

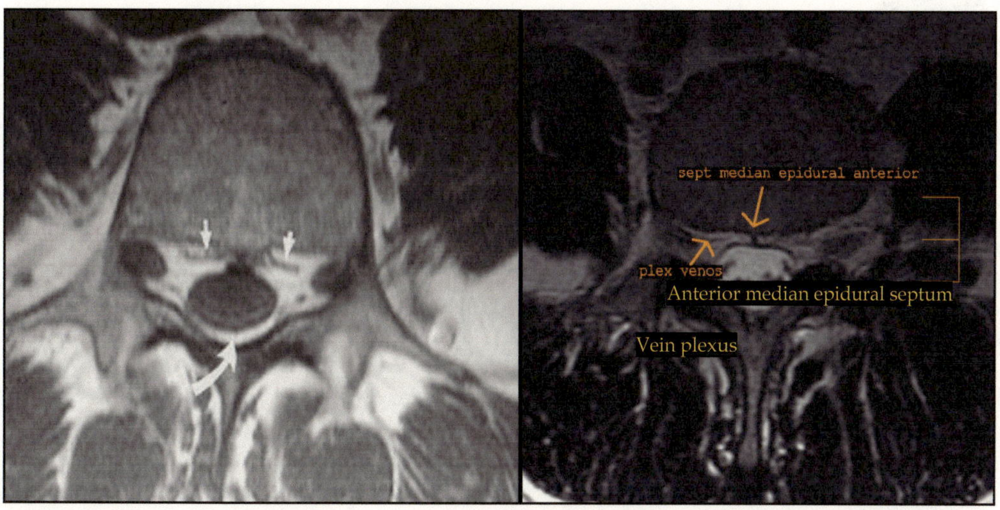

Fig. 10 a and b. Axial MRI section T1 and T2 through a lombar vertebra at the pediculo-lamar level. The fat in the epidural space is clearly visible, in hypersignal, surrounding the dural sac. The anterior vein plexuses can be well individualised (arrows). The posterior epidural space is somewhat poorly represented (curved arrow Figure a). Figure b - anterior median epidural septum

Our study has not emphasised any differences with regard to the time required for dilatation or the state of the foetus at the time of birth; however, the use of PCEA decreases the frequency and intensity of the engine block and reduces the need for an instrumental intervention, as the doses utilised are effective without there being a need to increase them.

The linearity of the VAS scale of quantifying pain varies between the two models, but the difference is statistically insignificant. (See Figure 11)

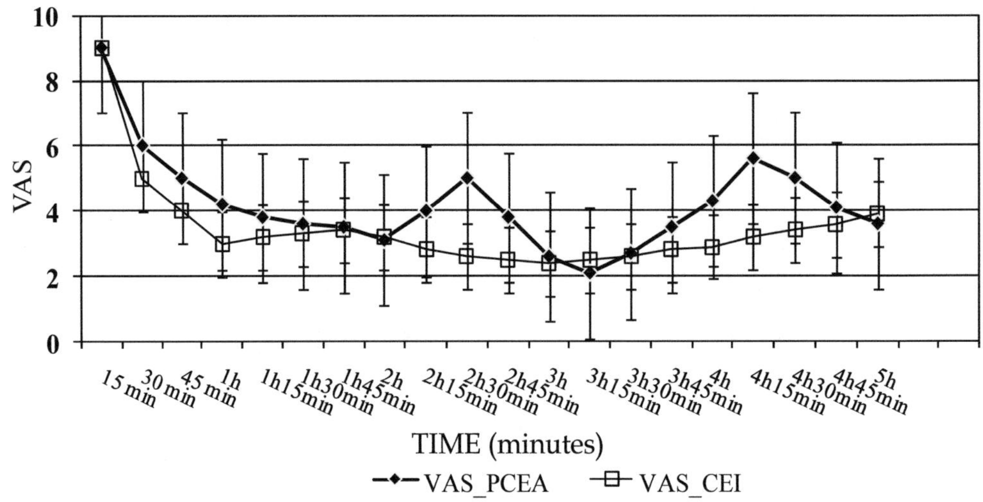

Fig. 11. VAS evolution in time, comparatively, in the two lots (p=NS)

CEI has ensured the decrease in frequency of the pain pick-ups on the VAS diagram during labour.

PCEA presents on the VAS diagram *pick-ups* corresponding to the increase in intensity of pain, which can be treated with the aid of the bolus doses placed at the disposal of the patient, without altering the high level of maternal satisfaction. The lack of a significant difference between the side effects of the two methods demonstrates the safety of the latter.

Although VAS linearity was maintained for CEI throughout labour, the analgesia at childbirth performed by means of the PCEA technique was appreciated by parturients, as they were their own deciders in controlling the pain.

In conclusion, although both techniques of epidural analgesia provide high maternal satisfaction, with a qualitatively good analgesia, PCEA offers the possibility to control pain while benefiting from the patient's collaboration. This simplifies the epidural analgesia protocol and decreases the number of invasive interventions from the part of the doctor. The technique ensures an individual calculation of the anaesthetic dose for an endurable degree of pain and decreases the number of instrumental interventions in the process of childbirth. Apart from these advantages, the absent or minimal motor block and the fall in the number of instrumental births using the PCEA technique are arguments worthy of taking into consideration in favour of this method.

4. PIEB

For the first time in Romania, we have conducted a transversal study, descriptively, by using a relatively new technique at the global level, namely epidural analgesia at childbirth through programmed boluses (PIEB - Programmed Intermittent Epidural Bolus), by which one can avoid high fluctuations of the sensorial levels attained, as it has been noticed in the case of PCEA, and reduce the total consumption of anaesthetic, compared to CEI.

We have included in our study a number of 28 parturients, ASA I, with a gestation age of over 37 weeks, and applied the epidural catheter at a dilatation of the cervix of 3-5 cm and regular uterine contractions at every 2-3 minutes. We have again used levobupivacaine with no additives as a local anaesthetic. Forty five minutes after the initial bolus of 10 ml of the 0,250 % solution, we have administered regular boluses of 6 ml from the 0,125% solution every 30 minutes until full dilatation.

Since in this study, the number of patients has been smaller (n=28) compared to CEI (n=53) and PCEA (n=41), the lots not being homogenous, we have not made a comparison between these lots, though including all the obstetrical parameters in the same table (See Table 6).

Parameters	**PIEB (n=28)**	**PCEA (n=41)***	**CEI (n=53) ***
Cervix dilatation at initiation of anesthesia (cm)	3.2 (3.1 - 3.3)	3.1 (3.1 - 3.2)	3.4 (3.1 - 3.7)
Duration of labour (min)	130 (120.5 - 142.22)	188.3 (180.3 - 196.4)	168.5 (162.2 - 174.8)
Motor block (n, %)	3 (10.71%)	2 (4.87%)	21 (39.7)
Maternal satisfaction	High	High	High
Childbirth by caesarean (n, %)	4 (14.28%)	4 (9.75%)	8 (15.09%)
Instrumental childbirth (vacuum extraction) (n, %)	1 (3.57%)	2 (2.12%)	14 (14.89%)

Table 6. Obstetrical parameters in patients who benefitted from PIEB, PCEA and CEI

As noticed, there are major differences between the PIEB lot and the CEI lot, but the results are similar between the PCEA and PIEB lots. We have found no differences between the PCEA and PIEB lots regarding the effectiveness of the anaesthetic substance, maternal satisfaction or side effects. Four (14,28%) parturients gave birth by caesarean due to malpresentation of foetuses (two of them had posterior rotation of the foetal occiput). In the case of a single pregnant woman it was necessary to have an instrumental childbirth. Posterior occipital rotation is frequent during labour, representing around 20% of all the positions at the beginning of labour and 5% of those at birth [Hess PE et al., 2000; Gardberg M et al., 1998]. These malpositions of the foetus increase the rate of childbirths by caesarean and instrumental interventions, prolonging the second stage of birth and causing perineal ruptures. There are authors who consider that epidural analgesia would favour the posterior rotation of the foetal occiput.

A study by Sebastiann *et al.* has shown that the regular use of programmed intermittent boluses could improve the function of the epidural catheter [American Society of Anesthesiologists Task Force on Obstetric Anesthesia, 2007]. Chua and Sia [Chua SM, Sia AT, 2004] have also noticed that PIEB represents a better alternative to childbirth analgesia than continuous perfusion.

We believe that analgesia at birth through programmed boluses is capable of ensuring rapid analgesia, extremely effective and with minimal motor block, low doses of local anaesthetic and increased maternal satisfaction (See Figure 12), thus it can rapidly become a widely utilised technique in alleviating pain [Dorca V et al., 2010].

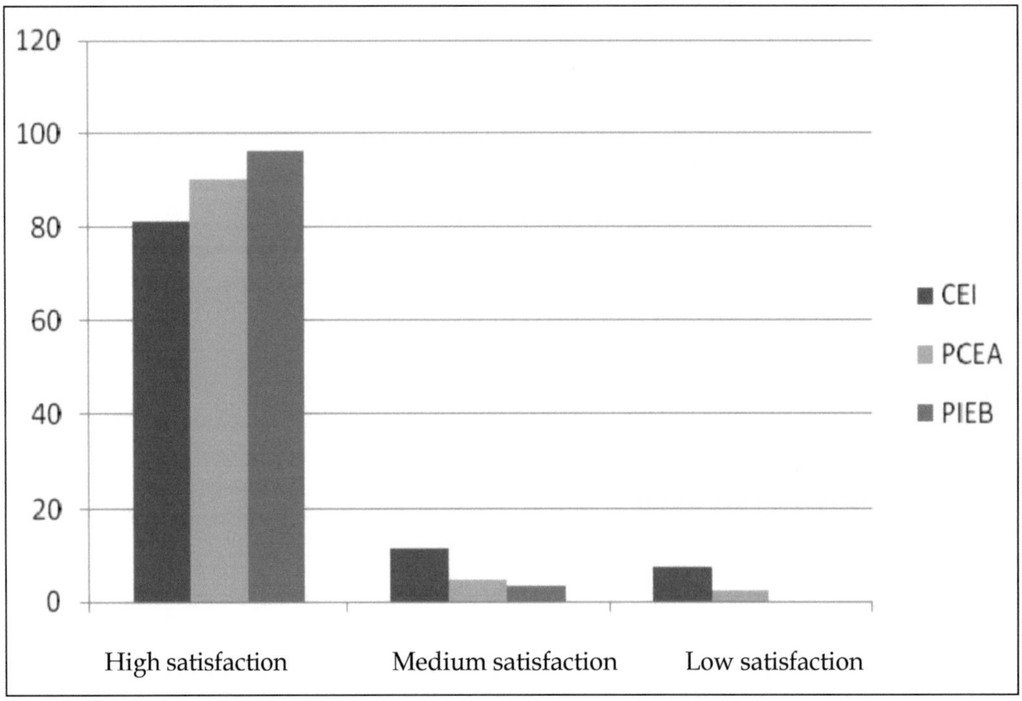

Fig. 12. Maternal satisfaction encountered in the three techniques utilised

In order to obtain rigorous results, it is necessary to conduct randomised studies which should validate this technique in the future. Since the infusion pumps that ensure a well-conducted analgesia through the PIEB technique are problematic [Sumikura H et al., 2004], it is our view that in the future, the technology incorporated into specialised electronic devices will solve this inconvenience.

5. Conclusion

The bolus injection of local anesthetic through an epidural catheter (PCEA/PIEB) has proven to be more efficient when considering the minimal intensity of motor blockade, the low local anesthetic consumption, the diminishing incidence of cesarean sections or instrumented deliveries and the parturient's satisfaction. However, in Romania, these techniques are not very popular yet.

Contrary to the developed countries, continuous epidural analgesia in labor is not very popular in Romania as a consequence of the lack of information among parturients.

6. References

Abboud T, Schnider S, Wright R. *Enflurane analgesia in obstetric*. Anesth Analg 1980; 60:133-137

Aggarwal A, Kaur H, Batra YK, Aggarwal AK, Rajeev S, Sahni D. *Anatomic consideration of caudal epidural space: A cadaver study*. Clin Anat. 2009 Jul 27

American Society of Anesthesiologists Task Force on Obstetric Anesthesia. *Practice guidelines for obstetric anesthesia*: an updated report by the American Society of Anesthesiologists Task Force on Obstetric Anesthesia. Anesthesiology 2007;106:843–63

Atherton MJ, Feeg VD, El-Adham AZ. *Race, ethnicity and insurance as determinants of epidural use*: analysis of a national sample survey. Nursing Economics. 2004;1:6-8.

Bonica J, Mc Donald JS. *Principles and Practice of Obstetric Analgesia and Anesthesia*. Williams & Wilkins, Malvern PA, USA; 2nd edition 1995; 344-537

Bromage P R, Burfoot M F, Ceowell D E. *Quality of epiduralblockade*. I. Influence of physical factors. Br J Anaesth 1964; 36: 342–352

Bussche EV, Crombez G, Eccleston C, Sullivan M. *Why women prefer epidural analgesia during childbirth: the role of beliefs about epidural analgesia and pain catastrophizing*. European Journal of Pain. 2007;11:275-282

Cathelin MF: *A new route of spinal injection: a method for epidural injection by way of the sacral canal: application to man*. Compt Rend Soc Biol 1901, 53:452

Chua SM, Sia AT. Automated intermittent epidural boluses improve analgesia induced by intrathecal fentanyl during labour. *Can J Anaesth*. 2004;51(6):581–585

Davidson EM, Sklar E, Bhatia R et al. *Magnetic Resonance Imaging Findings After Uneventful Continuous Infusion Neuraxial Analgesia: A Prospective Study to Determine Whether Epidural Infusion Produces Pathologic Magnetic Resonance Imaging Findings. Anesth Analg*. 2009 Jun 11

De Biasi P, Lupescu R, Burgun G et al. *Continuous lumbar plexus blocks: use of radiography to determine catheter tip location*. Reg Anesth Pain Med 2003; 28:135-9

Dogliotti AM. *A new method of block anesthesia: segmental peridural spinal anesthesia*. Am J Surg 1934; 20:107

Dorca V, Feier D, Groza D, Mihu D, Chiorean M. *Parturients' level of knowledge regarding labour analgesia in a university hospital- local exeprience*. Cj Med. 2011; 84 (1): 93-97

Dorca V, Feier D, Balintescu A, Belciu I, Groza D, Ciuchina S. *Analgezia periduralǎ cotrolatǎ de cǎtre pacientǎ comparativ cu infuzia periduralǎ continuǎ la naştere folosind levobupivacaina*. J Rom Anest Terap Int 2009; 16:99-106

Dorca V, Feier Diana, D. Mihu, C. Todea. *Programmed intermittent epidural bolus in labour: a cross-sectional study*. Acta Med Marisiensis. 2010; 56 (4): 370-372

El-Hamamy E, Arulkumaran S. *Poor progress of labour*. Current Obstetrics and Gynecology. 2005;1:1-8

Ferrante F M, Rosinia F A, Gordon C, Datta S. *The role of continuous background infusions in patient-controlled epidural analgesia for labor and delivery*. Anesth Analg 1994; 79: 80–84

Ferrante F M, Lu L, Jamison S B, Datta S. *Patient-controlled epidural analgesia: demand dosing. Anesth Analg 1991;* 73: 547–552

Gadalla F, Lee SH, Choi KC, Fong J, Gomillion MC, Leighton BL. *Injecting saline through the epidural needle decreases the iv epidural catheter placement rate during combined spinal-epidural labour analgesia.* Can J Anesth 2003; 50: 382–5

Gambling D R, Yu P, Cole C, McMorland G H, Palmer L. *A comparative study of patient controlled epidural analgesia (PCEA) and continuous infusion epidural analgesia (CIEA) during labour.* Can J Anaesth 1988; 35: 249–254

Gardberg M, Laakkonen E, Salevaara M. *Intrapartum sonography and persistent occiput posterior position: a study of 408 deliveries.* Obstet Gynecol 1998;91:746-9

Graffagnino P, Seyler LW. *Epidural anesthesia in obstetrics.* Am J Obstet Gynecol 1938; 35:597

Hess PE, Pratt SD, Soni AK, et al. *An association between severe labour pain and cesarean delivery.* Anesth Analg 2000;90:881–6

Lyons Gr, Kocarev MG, Wilson RC, Columb MO. *A comparison of minimum local anesthetic volumes and doses of epidural bupivacanie(0,125% w/v and 0,25% w/v) for analgesia in labor.* Anesth Analg 2007, 104: 412-5

Meister GC, D'Angelo R, Owen M, et al. *A comparison of epidural analgesia with 0.125% ropivacaine with fentanyl versus 0.125% bupivacaine with fentanyl during labor.* Anesth Analg 2000; 90:632–7

Minhas MR, Kamal R, Afshan G, Raheel H. *Knowledge, attitude and practice of parturients regarding epidural analgesia for labour in university hospital in Karachi.* The Journal of the Pakistan Medical Association. 2005;2:63-66.

Obst TE, Nauenberg E, Buck GM. *Maternal health insurance coverage as a determinant of obstetrical anesthesia care.* Journal of Health Care for the Poor and Underserved. 2001;12 (2):177-191

Owen MD, D'Angelo R, Gerancher JC, et al. *0.125% ropivacaine is similar to 0.125% bupivacaine for labor analgesia using patient-controlled epidural infusion.* Anesth Analg 1998;86: 527–31

Paech M. *Patient-controlled epidural analgesia.* In: Birnbach D J,Gatt S P, Datta S, eds. Textbook of Obstetric Anesthesia. 1.Philadelphia: Churchill Livingstone; 2000: 189–202

Robert R, Gaiser RR. *Labor epidurals and outcome (Best Practice and Research).* Clinical Anaesthesiology. 2005;1:1

Rust G, Nichols M, Omole F, Minor P, Barasso G, Mayberry R. *Racial and ethnic disparities in the provision of epidural analgesia to Georgia Medicaid beneficiaries during labor and delivery.* American Journal of Obstetrics and Gynecology. 2004;2:456-462

Salim R, Nachum Z, Moscovici R, Lavee M, Shalev E. *Continuous compared with intermittent epidural infusion on progress of labor and patient satisfaction.* Obstetrics and Gynaecology. 2005;2:301-306

Schlotterbeck H, Schaeffer R., Dow W.A. et al.: *Ultrasonographic control of the puncture level for lumbar neuraxial block in obstetric anesthesia.* Br J Anaesth 2008; 100:230–4

Sumikura H, van de Velde M, Tateda T. *Comparison between a disposable and an electronic PCA device for labour epidural analgesia.* J Anesth 2004;18:262–6

Van der Vyver M, Halpern S, Joseph G. *Patient-controlled epidural analgesia versus continuous infusion for labour analgesia: a metaanalysis.* Br J Anaesth 2002; 89: 459–465.

8

Combined Spinal Epidural Anesthesia and Analgesia

Dusica Stamenkovic[1] and Menelaos Karanikolas[2]
[1]*Department of Anesthesiology, Military Medical Academy, Belgrade,*
[2]*Department of Anesthesiology, Washington University School of Medicine, St. Louis,*
[1]*Serbia*
[2]*USA*

1. Introduction

In principle, the combination of two different administration of anesthesia routes on the same patient improves effectiveness and reduces side effects (Stevens and Edwards, 1999) [B]: Spinal anesthesia provides fast and reliable segmental anesthesia with minimal risk for toxicity, while epidural anesthesia provides perioperative anesthesia (alone or in combination with general anesthesia), followed by excellent analgesia in the postoperative period (Cook, 2000;Rawal et al., 2000) [A]. Moreover, Combined Spinal Epidural (CSE) anesthesia reduces the potential for problems, such as the somewhat unpredictable level of blockade after spinal anesthesia, and the problems of missed segments, incomplete motor block, poor sacral spread and local anesthetic toxicity that can occur with epidural anesthesia (Cook, 2000) [A]. At the present time, CSE anesthesia is widely used in orthopedic, urologic and gynecologic surgery. Major CSE anesthesia benefits are the need for low doses of medications, low incidence of motor blockade, adequate sensory block, the ability to extend the area of blockade if the surgical field needs to be extended, and excellent analgesia (Rawal et al., 1997) [A]. However, use of CSE anesthesia or analgesia also introduces the potential for complications, such as technical failure, altered spread of epidural drugs in patients who also had a lumbar puncture, and altered spread of subarachnoid medications due to the effects of the epidural injection.

2. History, anatomy, physiology and pharmacology

2.1 History

CSE anesthesia was first described in 1937 by Dr A. Soresi, an Italian surgeon who injected medications in the subarachnoid and epidural space at the same time (Brill et al., 2003;Waegerle, 1999). The procedure, as described by Dr Soresi, was called "Episubdural Anesthesia" and involved use of the same fine needle for both the epidural and the subarachnoid injection. The needle was first advanced in the epidural space using the hanging drop technique, and 8 ml of Novocain solution were injected. Then, the needle was advanced further, until it perforated the dura, and Novocain 2 ml was injected in the subarachnoid space (Cook, 2000). This CSE anesthesia study included over 200 patients and analgesia lasted for 24 to 48 hours (Soresi, 1937). Dr Soresi recommended that no preliminary medication should be given to allay fear, anxiety, or restlessness, because he strongly believed that sedatives make spinal and episubdural anesthesia unsafe, and stated in his paper that "to attempt to allay fear, anxiety and restlessness with any drug is to court disaster" (Soresi, 1937) [C]. Of note, the technique described by Dr Soresi was carried out in an era when there were no IV infusions (caffeine-containing saline or dextrose solutions were administered by epidermoclysis instead) and no monitoring capabilities. "Episubdural anesthesia" did not involve placement of an epidural catheter, and Dr Soresi concluded his paper stating that "the hanging drop method renders episubdural anesthesia the safest procedure giving perfect surgical anesthesia, ideal relaxation, and eliminating practically all postoperative pain and distress" (Soresi, 1937) [C].

Dr I. Curelaru was the first to publish a study on CSE anesthesia in 1979 in the German medical journal "Praktische Anasthesie Wiederbelebung und Intensivtherapie" (Brill et al., 2003). This study included 150 patients, and CSE anesthesia was performed in two different interspaces: First, the epidural catheter was placed; then, a subarachnoid injection of Dixidextracaine was carried out two levels below the level of epidural catheter insertion. Dr Curelaru concluded that CSE anesthesia confers several advantages, including high quality conduction anesthesia that could be extended as needed, prolonged postoperative analgesia, analgesia covering a satisfactory number of dermatomes, minimal local anesthetic toxicity and absence of pulmonary complications (Curelaru, 1979) [B]. In addition, Dr Curelaru also discussed the drawbacks of the technique, including the need for two lumbar punctures, prolonged procedural time for the double procedure, and difficulty locating the subarachnoid space after inserting a catheter in the epidural space. The same year, Dr Brownridge proposed using CSE anesthesia for Cesarean section, and published his results, two years later in "Anaesthesia" (Brownridge, 1981;Carrie, 1988). Then, in 1982, Dr Coates et al. and Dr Mumtaz et al. described a technical innovation, introducing the "needle through needle" technique: (Coates, 1982;Mumtaz et al., 1982) local anesthetic was first injected in the subarachnoid space, and this injection was followed by placement of an epidural catheter. The use of a special CSE needle set was reported for the first time by Carrie and O'Sullivan in 1984, in the "European Journal of Anaesthesiology" (Carrie and O'Sullivan, 1984). The use of CSE anesthesia in obstetrics was first reported in 1989 at the "Queen Charlotte" Hospital in London (Cook, 2000).

2.2 Anatomy and physiology

The epidural space, a potential space between the ligamentum flavum and the dura mater, surrounds the dural sac and contains fatty tissue and thin-walled blood vessels. The actual size of the epidural space varies: it is narrow in the thoracic region, due to spinal cord protuberances in the upper thoracic and bulges in the lower thoracic region, but it is wider below the level where the spinal cord ends (Katz and Renck, 1987). The distribution of epidural fat is also very important, because the course of the epidural catheter within the epidural space is influenced more by the epidural fat, rather than by connective tissue (Holmstrom et al., 1995). Because epidural fat is less viscous in children and more dense in adults, epidural catheters can be advanced more easily in children (Katz and Renck, 1987). Periduroscopic observations indicate that upon entering the epidural space, the epidural needle tip is in contact with the dura (Holmstrom et al., 1995). Therefore, variable further advancement of the spinal needle beyond the epidural needle tip is required in order to puncture the elastic dura when performing needle-through-needle CSE technique. The distance between the tip of the epidural needle and the posterior wall of the dural sac can be more than 10 mm in the midline; however, because the test injection used for identification of the epidural space may push the dura further back, the spinal needle used for CSE needs to be longer than conventional spinal needles (Rosenberg, 1998;Urmey, 2000). Consequently, CSE sets include extra long spinal needles, and it is important that CSE is performed caudad to the termination of the spinal cord at L2 (Katz and Renck, 1987).

2.3 Pharmacology

CSE anesthesia is an effective way to reduce drug doses required for anesthesia or analgesia, and the choice of medications is based on the concept of anti-nociceptive synergy: subarachnoid lipid soluble opioids (fentanyl or sufentanil) provide rapid (within 5-10 min) analgesia onset, improve surgical blockade quality (Rathmell et al., 2005) [A] and enhance the effect of small subarachnoid local anesthetic (bupivacaine) doses (Ben-David et al., 1997) [B], whereas subarachnoid morphine provides prolonged (lasting up to 24 hr) analgesia (Benzon HT et al., 2007). Furthermore, subarachnoid bupivacaine potentiates the effects of epidural bupivacaine (Stienstra et al., 1999) [B] and the anti-nociceptive effect of subarachnoid morphine (Akerman et al., 1988) [C].

The subarachnoid injection achieves rapid onset with minimal doses of local anesthetics and opioids, and the block can be prolonged as needed with low-doses of epidural medications. In addition, the sequential CSE method can be used to extend the dermatomal spread of the block with addition of minimal amounts of medications (Rawal, 2005;Rawal et al., 2000) [A]. The safety of CSE anesthesia is enhanced by the presence of the epidural catheter, which allows use of the lowest effective local anesthetic dose, thereby avoiding overshooting with regards to duration of spinal anesthesia. The rapid onset of anesthesia (from the spinal component) and the flexibility conferred by the epidural catheter make CSE anesthesia a safe and reliable anesthetic technique.

Reduction of drug doses with CSE anesthesia has made selective blockade possible, and many studies confirm that low-dose CSE anesthesia with local anesthetic and opioid, or low-dose epidural block alone, can provide effective analgesia with minimal motor and proprioceptive block. This selective blockade has made it possible for many patients to walk and bear weight normally while in labor and in the postoperative period. Therefore, CSE anesthesia is especially helpful for ambulatory surgical procedures of uncertain duration (Urmey, 2000), because the epidural catheter allows conversion from spinal to epidural anesthesia when it is necessary to extend the duration of the block. Of note, if the duration of surgery outlasts the initial subarachnoid block, it is necessary to inject at least 10 to 15 ml of local anesthetic through the epidural catheter in order to maintain satisfactory anesthesia (Urmey, 2000).

CSE anesthesia often produces a more extensive block than expected, and the epidural dose needed to extend the block is often lower compared to doses needed with epidural anesthesia alone (Lew et al., 2004;Rawal et al., 1988) [A]. This observation has two possible explanations (Stienstra et al., 1996;Stienstra et al., 1999). First, the alleviation of sub-atmospheric pressure by the Tuohy needle before injection of the local anesthetic can reduce the volume of the subarachnoid space in the dural sac and extend the level of spinal anesthesia (Felsby and Juelsgaard, 1995). Second, diffusion of local anesthetic molecules from the epidural to the subarachnoid space through the dural hole is possible, due to dural sac compression after injection of local anesthetic in the epidural space (Blumgart et al., 1992).

A randomized controlled trial (RCT) by Tyagi et al studied the dose-sparing effect of epidural volume extension by comparing the ED50 of plain vs. hyperbaric bupivacaine with and without epidural volume extension in 88 male patients undergoing lower extremity orthopedic surgery. This study showed that, compared to hyperbaric bupivacaine, plain bupivacaine appears to be more effective, requiring a smaller dose and producing a higher sensory block with earlier onset. It also showed that epidural volume extension, when applied to subarachnoid hyperbaric bupivacaine, does not decrease the dose of subarachnoid medication and does not raise the level of block (Tyagi et al., 2008).

Spinal block during CSE may produce more extensive spread of local anesthetic in the subarachnoid space, compared to spinal block with the single shot technique in women having cesarean section. If that is true, then a smaller dose of local anesthetic will achieve a similar level of block when the CSE technique is used (Ithnin et al., 2006). However, data from two recent RCTs contradict these findings, and suggest that, when comparing single-shot spinal vs. CSE anesthesia, equal subarachnoid anesthetic doses produce comparable level of sensory blockade, and there is no need for adjustment of subarachnoid doses (Horstman et al., 2009;Lim et al., 2006). Similarly, a study by Kucukguclu evaluated the effect of epidural volume extension in women undergoing cesarean section under spinal anesthesia using the CSE technique with hyperbaric vs. plain 0.5% bupivacaine. This study did not show an effect of epidural volume extension on the spread of spinal anesthesia (Kucukguclu et al., 2008).

Recommended doses for standard CSE anesthesia in non-obstetric surgery are bupivacaine or levobupivacaine 0.5% 12.5 to 20 mg, combined with preservative free morphine sulphate 100-300 µg for subarachnoid single shot injection (Rawal et al., 2000) [A]. Subarachnoid fentanyl (lipid-soluble, quick onset) and preservative-free morphine (water-soluble, slower onset, long duration) combined with small doses of subarachnoid bupivacaine can synergistically produce rapid and sustained analgesia (Gwirtz et al., 1999) [B]. Epidural top-ups require bupivacaine or levobupivacaine 0.5% 20-30 mg combined with fentanyl 25µg or sufentanil 2.5-5 µg (Bouvet et al., 2011) [B].

CSE for cesarean section requires subarachnoid bupivacaine 0.5-0.75%, 7.5-15 mg combined with opioids. Recommended opioid doses are fentanyl 20-25 µg and morphine 100-200 µg (somewhat lower compared to non obstetric patients). Epidural top-ups require bupivacaine or levobupivacaine 0.25 to 0.5% 10-40 mg combined with fentanyl 25µg or sufentanil 2.5-5 µg (Bouvet et al., 2011) [B]. Subarachnoid ropivacaine can also be used, but ropivacaine doses are 50% higher, compared to bupivacaine or levobupivacaine (Coppejans and Vercauteren, 2006) [B].

Sequential CSE anesthesia for cesarean section requires subarachnoid hyperbaric bupivacaine 0.5% 5-7.5 mg (the opioid dose is unchanged). Reduced subarachnoid hyperbaric bupivacaine doses result in adequate surgical analgesia with slower onset of maternal hypotension and decreased incidence of adverse effects. Epidural top-ups require bupivacaine 0.2-0.5% 10-50 mg with fentanyl 20-25 μg or sufentanil 5-10 μg. Similarly, studies in non-obstetric surgery show that when CSE anesthesia is performed in the sitting position, epidural volume extension does not decrease the dose or raise the level of block produced by subarachnoid hyperbaric bupivacaine (Beale et al., 2005;Rawal, 2005;Tyagi et al., 2008) [A].

A RCT on patients undergoing major orthopedic surgery under spinal levobupivacaine/ sufentanil anesthesia, supplemented by subarachnoid $MgSO_4$ (94.5 mg, 6.3%) and epidural $MgSO_4$ (2%, 100 mg/h) showed that subarachnoid and epidural magnesium significantly reduced patients' post-operative opioid analgesic requirements (Arcioni et al., 2007) [B].

3. Indications, contraindications and clinical use of CSE Anesthesia

Although CSE anesthesia was originally described for urologic surgery, indications for its use have expanded in recent years. CSE is now widely used in obstetrics (for labor analgesia and for cesarean sections), orthopedic surgery, trauma, abdominal, vascular and gynecologic surgery (Curelaru, 1979). CSE anesthesia allows the use of very low subarachnoid drug doses, due to the synergistic interaction between subarachnoid and epidural drugs. The CSE anesthesia is very appropriate for outpatient surgery, because the block wears off rapidly, so that patients ambulate earlier and can be discharged home sooner (Urmey, 2000;Urmey et al., 1995;Urmey et al., 1996) [B]. Contraindications to CSE anesthesia are the same as for any neuraxial block.

Surgery type	Surgical procedure
Obstetrics	Labor analgesia, Cesarean Section
Gynecology	Hysterectomy
Orthopedics	Hip and knee surgery
Urology	Prostatectomy, cystectomy
Abdominal surgery	Colorectal, renal transplantation
Vascular surgery	Open surgical repair of infrarenal abdominal aortic aneurysm Reconstructive surgery of lower extremities
Ambulatory surgery	Knee arthroscopy
Pediatric surgery	Abdominal surgery

Table 1. Use of CSE anesthesia in surgical practice

4. CSE Techniques

4.1 Needle-through-needle technique

The first "spinal-needle-through-epidural needle" technique was described by Coates (Rosenberg, 1998). After the epidural space is identified using an epidural needle, the epidural needle serves as introducer, and a fine spinal needle is advanced through the epidural needle, beyond its tip, until it punctures the dura. Medications are first injected in the subarachnoid space, and then the epidural catheter is inserted. Disadvantages of this technique are the possibility for advancing the epidural catheter into the subarachnoid space, and the possibility for needle damage from friction between the needles. Although it is possible to combine a plain Tuohy needle with a longer, thinner spinal needle for performing the procedure, special commercial "all in one" kits have become available. Long thin needles make it more difficult to feel perforation of the dura; therefore, the "hanging drop" technique is recommended to identify the spinal space after dura perforation (Kopacz and Bainton, 1996) [C].The "Hanging drop" technique consists of placing one drop of normal saline in the hub of spinal needle. This "hanging drop" will fall down from the hub of the needle when the spinal needle reaches the subarachnoid space.

"Backeye" is the hole constructed in the curvature of the epidural needle tip, so that the spinal needle can advance along a straight route into the epidural space. This design allows smooth advancement of the spinal needle, without friction between the epidural catheter and the spinal needle, and may reduce the risk of epidural catheter migration through holes opened by the spinal needle (Hanaoka K, 1986;Liu and McDonald, 2001) [B].

The Espocan CSE set (Braun) contains an epidural needle constructed with a plastic sleeve inside. This sleeve leads the spinal needle and separates it from the epidural catheter (Browne et al., 2005). Information on this set is available online. Another commercial product, the Epistar needle, has two channels: one for the epidural catheter and one for the spinal needle. The Epistar needle confers the advantage that spinal anesthesia is performed after the epidural catheter has been inserted and a test dose has been given to confirm proper epidural catheter placement. (Stamenkovic et al., 2009) [B]. Information on the Epistar CSE set is also available online.

4.2 Separate needles

In this technique, the two components of CSE (spinal and epidural injection) are performed using separate needles, in the same or at different inter-vertebral spaces, in either order (Cook, 2000).

Performing both the epidural and spinal injection at the same interspace requires infiltration with local anesthetic only once. When using this technique, the epidural needle is placed first, to serve as introducer for the spinal needle at the same interspace. Then, after the epidural catheter is advanced, the spinal needle is advanced in order to puncture the dura and allow the subarachnoid injection (Turner and Reifenberg, 1995) [B]. When using this technique, epidural catheter damage caused with spinal needle during dural puncture is a possible complication. A modification of this technique, proposed by Cook, suggested that the spinal needle be placed as low as possible in the interspace, whereas the epidural catheter be placed cephalad, and then subarachnoid injection be performed (Cook, 2004) [B].

The technique using two different interspaces confers the advantage that it allows epidural catheter placement in the thoracic or the lumbar area, depending on the location of the pain, while the subarachnoid injection is still done in the lumbar area (Stamenkovic et al., 2008) [B]. In addition, this technique allows the use of an epidural test dose to confirm appropriate placement of the epidural catheter before the spinal injection, and avoids potential puncture of the epidural catheter by the spinal needle. However, despite these presumed advantages, in the absence of robust evidence, expert opinion suggests that, compared to the separate interspaces technique, the "needle-through-needle" technique causes "considerably less discomfort, trauma and morbidity from inter-spinous space penetration including backache, epidural venous puncture, hematoma, infection and technical difficulties" (Rawal et al., 1997).

4.3 Special single CSE needles

The Eldor needle technique is a slightly different technique that was introduced in 1990, and uses a specialized needle for CSE. The Eldor needle is both spinal and epidural needle, combining an 18G epidural needle with a 20G spinal conduit, and the epidural catheter can be introduced before the spinal injection. An image of the needle is available online at the company website. Use of the Eldor needle reduces the risk of accidental subarachnoid placement of the epidural catheter, and avoids friction of the needles and post-dural puncture headaches. The Eldor needle is used as follows: First, the spinal needle is introduced into the guide needle. Then, the Eldor needle is placed in the selected inter-vertebral space, using the "loss of resistance" technique to locate the epidural space. After reaching the epidural space, the epidural catheter is inserted first, and then the spinal needle is advanced until it perforates the dura. Following the subarachnoid injection, the spinal needle is removed, and then the Eldor needle is also removed.

The Coombs epidural –spinal needle is a newer multi-lumen device (Eldor, 1997) that has two different channels, with the spinal channel being underneath the epidural channel. However, despite their advantages, Eldor needles and Coombs needles have not gained widespread popularity because they are uncomfortably large (Rosenberg, 1998) [B].

A RCT comparing a CSE set with an interlocking device between the spinal and epidural needle vs. a CSE set with a "backeye" at the epidural needle curve for passage of the spinal needle vs. the double-segment technique, showed that use of CSE sets does not save time compared with the double segment technique (Puolakka et al., 2001). Moreover damaged spinal needle tips were noted relatively often with the interlocking CSE set [B].

4.4 Dual catheter technique

The dual catheter technique involves the insertion of two catheters, one in the epidural space and one in the subarachnoid space on the same patient. Having both an epidural and a subarachnoid catheter confers certain advantages, in that both spinal anesthesia and epidural analgesia can be extended or prolonged, as needed for surgery and postoperative analgesia. However, having two similar catheters on the same patient introduces the potential for serious errors, mainly the inadvertent subarachnoid injection of medications in doses intended for epidural use. Clearly, such errors could be life-threatening if not detected early. At the present time due to concerns about the risk of inadvertent epidural injection of local anesthetic through the subarachnoid, rather than through the epidural catheter, the dual catheter technique is rarely used (Dahl et al., 1990;Vercauteren et al., 1993).

5. Comparison of CSE vs. spinal or epidural anesthesia or analgesia

Compared to conventional neuraxial (spinal or epidural) anesthesia, CSE anesthesia is technically more demanding, but can confer certain advantages. Data on proven or potential advantages of CSE anesthesia compared to epidural or spinal anesthesia are as follows:

A RCT on 75 patients undergoing major orthopedic surgery compared CSE vs. spinal vs. epidural anesthesia, and showed that spinal and CSE provided effective and reliable block with muscle relaxation and good surgical conditions rapidly, and both techniques were superior to epidural anesthesia (Holmstrom et al., 1993) [B].

A retrospective chart review in a community hospital assessed the safety and efficacy of 6,002 CSE analgesia/anesthesia blocks, and compared these results with reported complications and failure rates for spinal and epidural anesthesia. This study showed that, compared to epidural anesthesia, CSE anesthesia had lower failure rates for labor analgesia and comparable or lower failure rates for surgical anesthesia. There were no cases of apnea among parturients who received 4,164 CSE blocks with subarachnoid sufentanil (10, 15, or 20 μg) for labor analgesia. However, the need for intravenous medications to treat CSE side-effects increased with increasing subarachnoid sufentanil doses: medications were needed in 1.1% of patients who received sufentanil 10 μg, 4.6% of patients who received sufentanil 15 μg, and 5.5% of patients who received sufentanil 20 μg. The study concluded that CSE was safe and efficacious for labor and surgical anesthesia (Albright and Forster, 1999) [B].

Use of CSE anesthesia or epidural improved postoperative recovery in patients undergoing retro-pubic prostatectomy, and resulted in one day hospitalization with minimal postoperative morbidity and high patient satisfaction (Kirsh et al., 2000) [B].

Furthermore, CSE anesthesia was performed in the right lateral position using a double-space technique in 50 patients undergoing renal transplantation. Neuraxial blockade was satisfactory in all but four patients who required supplemental general anesthesia for prolonged surgery. This study concluded that CSE anesthesia was very useful, combining the reliability of spinal block with the versatility of epidural block for renal transplantation (Bhosale and Shah, 2008) [B]. CSE anesthesia can also be safely used for living donor nephrectomy, resulting in good surgeon satisfaction and patient comfort, and could be the method of choice for patients anxious about general anesthesia (Haberal et al., 2002) [C].

Postoperative pain after abdominal surgery (especially surgery involving more than one organ) is a challenge in institutions where expensive delivery systems, such as infusion pumps for continuous epidural analgesia, are not available. Compared to epidural analgesia, CSE analgesia using preoperative subarachnoid morphine, fentanyl and bupivacaine resulted in better postoperative control of pain with cough, fewer additional analgesia requests in the first 24 hours postoperatively, and reduced amounts of supplemental intra-operative IV fentanyl and epidural bupivacaine (Stamenkovic et al., 2008) [B].

6. CSE anesthesia in special populations

6.1 Patients with significant cardiac or pulmonary disease

CSE anesthesia alone, without general anesthesia, intubation or mechanical ventilation, can be a good anesthetic option in patients with severe chronic obstructive pulmonary disease (COPD) who undergo open repair of infra-renal abdominal aortic aneurysm (AAA), if general anesthesia would pose too high a risk and endovascular repair is not feasible (Berardi et al., 2010) [C]. Berardi et al, presented series of seven high-risk patients ages 70 to 87 undergoing open AAA repair. Average AAA diameter was 7 cm (range 6-12.2). The anesthetic plan included spinal anesthesia at L2-3 (levobupivacaine plus fentanyl), combined with epidural anesthesia at T7-8 (levobupivacaine). All patients tolerated the procedure well, without morbidity or mortality for 12 months after surgery.

Another case series described three patients undergoing open infrarenal AAA repair under CSE anesthesia, and concluded that CSE anesthesia is a "viable" anesthetic option in patients with severe COPD, because it can preserve spontaneous breathing and provide respiratory benefits over general anesthesia (Flores et al., 2002) [C].

Use of CSE anesthesia has also been reported in patients with severe COPD undergoing abdominoplasty, sigmoid-colectomy, right hemicolectomy and cholecystectomy (Kodeih et al., 2009;Moiniche et al., 1994;Morton and Bowler, 2001;van Zundert et al., 2007).

The safety of low-dose sequential CSE analgesia in women with unrepaired cyanotic heart disease who required analgesia for labor has recently been reported (Arendt et al., 2011) [C]. In addition, one case report described successful management of a patient with untreated ventricular septal defect and pulmonary atresia who had hysterectomy under CSE anesthesia (Agarwal et al., 2010).

6.2 CSE anesthesia in the elderly

Several studies have investigated the use of CSE anesthesia in geriatric patients. One study from Japan on 17 patients older than 80 years who underwent lower extremity orthopedic surgery showed that, compared to spinal or epidural anesthesia alone, CSE anesthesia was preferred, providing rapid onset, reliable spinal block and high quality intraoperative and postoperative analgesia (Wakamatsu et al., 1991). Another study by Tahtaci et al. on 19 elderly patients (mean age 75.8 years) showed that CSE anesthesia provides "sufficient anaesthesia with fewer complications" than spinal anesthesia (Tahtaci and Neyal, 2002) [C].

Similarly, a case report by Morton described the successful use of CSE anesthesia for sigmoid colectomy in an 82-year-old woman with congestive heart disease, COPD, osteoporosis and severe kyphosis (Morton and Bowler, 2001).

6.3 CSE anesthesia in obstetrics

Because traditional epidural techniques have been associated with prolonged labor, increased need for oxytocin augmentation, and increased incidence of instrumental vaginal delivery, CSE was introduced in obstetrics as an attempt to reduce these adverse effects. CSE is currently very popular in obstetric anesthesia and analgesia (Blanshard and Cook, 2004), because it is believed to improve maternal mobility during labor and, compared to traditional epidural analgesia, provide more rapid onset of analgesia and higher maternal satisfaction. In addition, CSE allows prolongation of epidural analgesia or conversion to CSE anesthesia, if cesarean section is needed.

A retrospective study on 77 pre-eclamptic parturients (26 women with severe pre-eclampsia, 51 with mild pre-eclampsia) undergoing Cesarean section, showed that CSE anesthesia is safe in women with pre-eclampsia and severe pre-eclampsia (Van, V et al., 2004) [B].

In addition, CSE can be a good option in pregnant women with a variety of serious medical conditions: CSE anesthesia or analgesia was successfully used in a parturient with severe myasthenia gravis (D'Angelo and Gerancher, 1998), idiopathic hypertrophic sub-aortic stenosis (Ho et al., 1997), mitral stenosis (Ngan Kee et al., 1999), dilated cardiomyopathy (Shnaider et al., 2001), Guillain-Barre syndrome (Vassiliev et al., 2001), Laron syndrome (Bhatia and Cockerham, 2011), tetralogy of Fallot (Arendt et al., 2011), Liddle's syndrome (Hayes et al., 2011), Wegener's granulomatosis with subglottic stenosis (Engel et al., 2011).

Another prospective study on 2183 laboring women, showed that labor progress and outcome are similar among women receiving either CSE or epidural analgesia and that CSE analgesia is not associated with increased frequency of anesthetic complications (Norris et al., 2001) [B].

A Cochrane review analyzed nineteen trials (2658 women) evaluating CSE vs. epidural analgesia in labor (Simmons et al., 2007) [A]. Twenty-six outcomes in two sets of comparisons involving CSE vs. traditional epidurals and CSE vs. low-dose epidural techniques were analyzed. When comparing CSE vs. traditional epidural analgesia, CSE was better with regards to need for rescue analgesia and urinary retention, but was associated with more pruritus. When comparing CSE vs. low-dose epidurals, CSE patients experienced faster onset of effective analgesia, but more pruritus. In addition, CSE was associated with lower (not clinically significant) umbilical arterial pH, but there were no differences with regards to maternal satisfaction, mobilization during labor, maternal hypotension, modes of birth, incidence of post-dural puncture headache or need for epidural blood patch. It was not possible to draw any conclusions regarding maternal respiratory depression, maternal sedation and need for augmentation of labor, and there was no difference in obstetric or neonatal outcomes. Based on these results, the authors concluded that available evidence cannot support a specific recommendation for CSE vs. epidurals in labor. However, the significantly higher incidence of urinary retention and rescue interventions needed with traditional epidurals would favor the use of low-dose epidurals. Currently available data cannot support any conclusions regarding rare complications such as nerve injury or meningitis.

6.4 CSE anesthesia in pediatrics

In order to evaluate the safety of CSE anesthesia in neonates and infants undergoing elective major abdominal surgery, spinal anesthesia was performed in 28 neonates and infants using isobaric bupivacaine 0.5%, 1 mg/kg, followed by placement of a caudal epidural catheter that was advanced to reach thoracic spinal segments (Somri et al., 2007). This study showed that CSE was well tolerated, and the authors concluded that "CSE anesthesia could be considered as an effective anesthetic technique for elective major upper abdominal surgery in awake or sedated neonates and infants, and could be used cautiously by a pediatric anesthesiologist as an alternate to general anesthesia in high-risk neonates and infants undergoing upper gastrointestinal surgery". However, four patients required conversion from CSE anesthesia to general anesthesia, whereas twenty patients required midazolam for sedation, oxygen supplementation and transient manual ventilation.

One more study included 19 infants undergoing major abdominal surgery (including small bowel resections and genitourinary procedures) under CSE anesthesia with spinal tetracaine and epidural bupivacaine. Then, epidural analgesia was successfully used for postoperative pain (Williams et al., 1997).

Fifty infants undergoing elective gastrointestinal surgery were included in a RCT designed to compare CSE vs. general anesthesia with regards to cardio-respiratory adverse events during an 8-day follow-up period in the intensive care unit (Somri et al., 2011). This study showed that, compared to patients receiving general anesthesia, patients who received CSE anesthesia had fewer adverse respiratory and cardiovascular events [B]. Furthermore, adverse cardiovascular events were more resistant to treatment in the general anesthesia group.

In conclusion, limited data suggest that CSE can be very useful in certain pediatric surgery patients. However, more research is needed to fully evaluate the role of CSE in pediatric surgery.

7. Concerns, technical failures and potential complications of CSE anesthesia

Potential concerns related to the clinical use of CSE include failure of the spinal and/or epidural component, spinal migration of the epidural catheter, the possibility of subdural block and the potential for subarachnoid administration of medications intended for epidural use. Other potential problems include failure of the test dose, post-dural puncture headache, and very rare catastrophic complications, including CNS injuries or CNS infection.

7.1 Epidural catheter migration into the subarachnoid space

The possibility that the epidural catheter could migrate into the subarachnoid space through the hole created on the dura by the spinal needle is subject to controversy. Published data suggest that rotation of the epidural needle is unnecessary, because there is no risk for epidural dislodgement into the subarachnoid space, if the dural puncture is performed with a 26-gauge spinal needle (Rawal et al., 1988). However, it is still possible that epidurally administered medications could enter the subarachnoid space through the hole in dura, especially if "wet tap" occurred (Bernards et al., 1994).

7.2 Failure of the spinal or epidural component of CSE

Some data suggest that failure rate of the spinal component of CSE (approximately 5%) is higher compared to spinal anesthesia alone (Cook, 2000). Indeed, there are several reasons why the spinal component could fail more frequently during CSE. First, the small size of the spinal needle can contribute to failure, because the thinner, smaller spinal needles used for CSE result in slower return of cerebrospinal fluid (CSF) and higher resistance to injection (Liu and McDonald, 2001). Second, movement of the spinal needle beyond the epidural needle can be problematic when the tiny spinal needle loses support. Third, deviation of the spinal needle away from midline is a possibility that could compromise success of the subarachnoid injection (Rawal et al., 1997). In addition, if water is used for the "loss of resistance" technique during epidural placement, water return through the hub of the spinal needle can be wrongly interpreted as CSF (Liu and McDonald, 2001).

The epidural component of CSE can also fail: If the subarachnoid injection is performed before the epidural block, use of a test dose to confirm appropriate epidural catheter placement is no longer possible. The incidence of failure of the epidural CSE component is unknown (Liu and McDonald, 2001), but, unfortunately epidural block failure can only be recognized late, after surgery has started.

7.3 Paresthesias

During CSE, paresthesias occur at the time of spinal needle advancement in 2.6% to 10% of cases, but the incidence has been reported to be up to 29% when long spinal needles are used (Casati et al., 1998;Herbstman et al., 1998;Hoffmann et al., 1997). Long needles, particularly when the length beyond the tip of the epidural needle was longer than 12 mm, caused more transitional paresthesia during needle insertion, but no residual effects (Herbstman et al., 1998). One case of prolonged left lower limb paresis has been reported following CSE anesthesia for obstetric surgery. Magnetic resonance imaging (MRI) in this case showed marked swelling of the lower end of the spinal cord suggesting traumatic damage of the cord by the spinal needle (Rajakulendran et al., 1999).

7.4 Cauda equina syndrome

Two cases of cauda equina syndrome have been reported after CSE (Kubina et al., 1997). In another case, the patient reported buttock numbness with an area of hypesthesia in the distribution of the lower sacral nerves, but there were no significant imaging findings, and sensation fully recovered after 7 months (Paech, 1997). The etiology of neurologic deficits in these cases remains unknown, but drug-induced neurotoxicity could be a plausible explanation.

7.5 Meningitis

The risk of meningitis after CSE is unknown, but several cases of aseptic or bacterial post CSE meningitis have been reported with the needle-through-needle or the two space technique (Aldebert and Sleth, 1996;Harding et al., 1994;Kasai et al., 2003;Sandkovsky et al., 2009;Vasquez et al., 2002). Meticulous aseptic technique is important during CSE, and special care is needed to maintain sterility while preparing drug solutions (Rawal et al., 2000).

7.6 Epidural abscess

Although epidural abscess is rare, two case reports have described epidural abscess formation after CSE (Dysart and Balakrishnan, 1997;Schroter et al., 1997). One of these two patients was managed conservatively (Dysart and Balakrishnan, 1997), while the other patient required hemi-laminectomy and surgical drainage of the abscess (Schroter et al., 1997).

7.7 Adhesive arachnoiditis

Recently, Hirai et al published an extremely rare case of paraplegia due to adhesive arachnoiditis with extensive syringomyelia (ES) and a giant anterior arachnoid spinal cyst (AASC) after CSE anesthesia for obstetric surgery in a young patient (Hirai et al., 2011). Spinal cord MRI showed spinal cord compression at T1-6 and an adhesive lesion at T7.

Posterior laminectomy at T6-7 and adhesiolysis of the arachnoid adhesion at T7 were performed, followed by cyst-peritoneal shunt into the AASC.

7.8 Subdural hematoma

One case of subdural hematoma has been reported after needle through needle CSE in an obstetric patient with mild thrombocytopenia (Bougher and Ramage, 1995).

8. Conclusion

CSE is the combination of spinal and epidural anesthesia and analgesia on the same patient. Compared to conventional spinal or epidural anesthesia, CSE is a newer technique that was developed in an attempt to combine the advantages of spinal and epidural anesthesia/analgesia, while minimizing their disadvantages. CSE is currently popular and it is used in a wide variety of clinical settings, including general surgery, vascular surgery, urology, orthopedic surgery, obstetrics and gynecology and pediatric surgery. CSE seems to be particularly useful in ambulatory surgery, because it facilitates early patient ambulation and discharge to home. In addition, CSE probably has a role in patients with significant co-morbidities, who need to undergo surgery and are considered at high risk for general anesthesia.

9. Clinical pearls

CSE consists of a single subarachnoid injection combined with insertion of an epidural catheter for intermittent or continuous epidural administration of medications

CSE is an effective way to reduce drug doses required for anesthesia and analgesia

CSE is safe and efficacious for labor analgesia and surgical anesthesia, particularly for ambulatory surgery

CSE anesthesia alone, without general anesthesia, can be a good anesthetic option in patients with severe chronic pulmonary disease

Low-dose sequential CSE anesthesia has been successfully used in adults with unrepaired cyanotic heart disease or other significant cardiac co-morbidities

Limited data suggest that CSE can be very useful in certain pediatric surgery patients

10. References

Agarwal, A., R. Garg, A. Joshi, and S. Verma, 2010, Combined spinal epidural anesthesia with epidural volume extension technique for hysterectomy in patient with unpalliated cyanotic heart disease--a case-report: Acta Anaesthesiol.Belg., v. 61, no. 3, p. 159-161.

Akerman, B., E. Arwestrom, and C. Post, 1988, Local anesthetics potentiate spinal morphine antinociception: Anesth.Analg., v. 67, no. 10, p. 943-948.

Albright, G. A., and R. M. Forster, 1999, The safety and efficacy of combined spinal and epidural analgesia/anesthesia (6,002 blocks) in a community hospital: Reg Anesth.Pain Med., v. 24, no. 2, p. 117-125.

Aldebert, S., and J. C. Sleth, 1996, [Bacterial meningitis after combined spinal and epidural anesthesia in obstetrics]: Ann.Fr.Anesth.Reanim., v. 15, no. 5, p. 687-688.

Arcioni, R. et al., 2007, Combined intrathecal and epidural magnesium sulfate supplementation of spinal anesthesia to reduce post-operative analgesic requirements: a prospective, randomized, double-blind, controlled trial in patients undergoing major orthopedic surgery: Acta Anaesthesiol.Scand., v. 51, no. 4, p. 482-489.

Arendt, K. W., S. M. Fernandes, P. Khairy, C. A. Warnes, C. H. Rose, M. J. Landzberg, P. A. Craigo, and J. R. Hebl, 2011, A case series of the anesthetic management of parturients with surgically repaired tetralogy of Fallot: Anesth.Analg., v. 113, no. 2, p. 307-317.

Beale, N., B. Evans, F. Plaat, M. O. Columb, G. Lyons, and G. M. Stocks, 2005, Effect of epidural volume extension on dose requirement of intrathecal hyperbaric bupivacaine at Caesarean section: Br.J.Anaesth., v. 95, no. 4, p. 500-503.

Ben-David, B., E. Solomon, H. Levin, H. Admoni, and Z. Goldik, 1997, Intrathecal fentanyl with small-dose dilute bupivacaine: better anesthesia without prolonging recovery: Anesth.Analg., v. 85, no. 3, p. 560-565.

Benzon HT, Candido KD, and Wong CA, 2007, Postoperative neuraxial analgesia, in Wong CA ed., Spinal and Epidural Anesthesia: New York, McGraw-Hill Companies Inc, p. 325-347.

Berardi, G. et al., 2010, Combined spinal and epidural anesthesia for open abdominal aortic aneurysm surgery in vigil patients with severe chronic obstructive pulmonary disease ineligible for endovascular aneurysm repair. Analysis of results and description of the technique: Int.Angiol., v. 29, no. 3, p. 278-283.

Bernards, C. M., D. J. Kopacz, and M. Z. Michel, 1994, Effect of needle puncture on morphine and lidocaine flux through the spinal meninges of the monkey in vitro. Implications for combined spinal-epidural anesthesia: Anesthesiology, v. 80, no. 4, p. 853-858.

Bhatia, K., and R. Cockerham, 2011, Anaesthetic management of a parturient with Laron syndrome: Int.J.Obstet.Anesth..

Bhosale, G., and V. Shah, 2008, Combined spinal-epidural anesthesia for renal transplantation: Transplant.Proc., v. 40, no. 4, p. 1122-1124.

Blanshard, H. J., and T. M. Cook, 2004, Use of combined spinal-epidural by obstetric anaesthetists: Anaesthesia, v. 59, no. 9, p. 922-923.

Blumgart, C. H., D. Ryall, B. Dennison, and L. M. Thompson-Hill, 1992, Mechanism of extension of spinal anaesthesia by extradural injection of local anaesthetic: Br.J.Anaesth., v. 69, no. 5, p. 457-460.

Bougher, R. J., and D. Ramage, 1995, Spinal subdural haematoma following combined spinal-epidural anaesthesia: Anaesth.Intensive Care, v. 23, no. 1, p. 111-113.

Bouvet, L., X. Da-Col, D. Chassard, F. Dalery, L. Ruynat, B. Allaouchiche, E. Dantony, and E. Boselli, 2011, ED and ED of intrathecal levobupivacaine with opioids for Caesarean delivery: Br.J.Anaesth., v. 106, no. 2, p. 215-220.

Brill, S., G. M. Gurman, and A. Fisher, 2003, A history of neuraxial administration of local analgesics and opioids: Eur.J.Anaesthesiol., v. 20, no. 9, p. 682-689.

Browne, I. M., D. J. Birnbach, D. J. Stein, D. A. O'Gorman, and M. Kuroda, 2005, A comparison of Espocan and Tuohy needles for the combined spinal-epidural technique for labor analgesia: Anesth.Analg., v. 101, no. 2, p. 535-40, table.

Brownridge, P., 1981, Epidural and subarachnoid analgesia for elective caesarean section: Anaesthesia, v. 36, no. 1, p. 70.

Carrie, L. E., 1988, Epidural versus combined spinal epidural block for caesarean section: Acta Anaesthesiol.Scand., v. 32, no. 7, p. 595-596.

Carrie, L. E., and G. O'Sullivan, 1984, Subarachnoid bupivacaine 0.5% for caesarean section: Eur.J.Anaesthesiol., v. 1, no. 3, p. 275-283.

Casati, A., A. D'Ambrosio, N. P. De, G. Fanelli, V. Tagariello, and F. Tarantino, 1998, A clinical comparison between needle-through-needle and double-segment techniques for combined spinal and epidural anesthesia: Reg Anesth.Pain Med., v. 23, no. 4, p. 390-394.

Coates, M. B., 1982, Combined subarachnoid and epidural techniques: Anaesthesia, v. 37, no. 1, p. 89-90.

Cook, T. M., 2000, Combined spinal-epidural techniques: Anaesthesia, v. 55, no. 1, p. 42-64.

Cook, T. M., 2004, 201 combined spinal-epidurals for anaesthesia using a separate needle technique: Eur.J.Anaesthesiol., v. 21, no. 9, p. 679-683.

Coppejans, H. C., and M. P. Vercauteren, 2006, Low-dose combined spinal-epidural anesthesia for cesarean delivery: a comparison of three plain local anesthetics: Acta Anaesthesiol.Belg., v. 57, no. 1, p. 39-43.

Curelaru, I., 1979, Long duration subarachnoid anaesthesia with continuous epidural block: Prakt.Anaesth., v. 14, no. 1, p. 71-78.

D'Angelo, R., and J. C. Gerancher, 1998, Combined spinal and epidural analgesia in a parturient with severe myasthenia gravis: Reg Anesth.Pain Med., v. 23, no. 2, p. 201-203.

Dahl, J. B., J. Rosenberg, W. E. Dirkes, T. Mogensen, and H. Kehlet, 1990, Prevention of postoperative pain by balanced analgesia: Br.J.Anaesth., v. 64, no. 4, p. 518-520.

Dysart, R. H., and V. Balakrishnan, 1997, Conservative management of extradural abscess complicating spinal-extradural anaesthesia for caesarean section: Br.J.Anaesth., v. 78, no. 5, p. 591-593.

Eldor, J., 1997, The evolution of combined spinal-epidural anesthesia needles: Reg Anesth., v. 22, no. 3, p. 294-296.

Engel, N. M., H. F. Gramke, L. Peeters, and M. A. Marcus, 2011, Combined spinal-epidural anaesthesia for a woman with Wegener's granulomatosis with subglottic stenosis: Int.J.Obstet.Anesth., v. 20, no. 1, p. 94-95.

Felsby, S., and P. Juelsgaard, 1995, Combined spinal and epidural anesthesia: Anesth.Analg., v. 80, no. 4, p. 821-826.

Flores, J. A., T. Nishibe, M. Koyama, T. Imai, F. Kudo, K. Miyazaki, and K. Yasuda, 2002, Combined spinal and epidural anesthesia for abdominal aortic aneurysm surgery in patients with severe chronic pulmonary obstructive disease: Int.Angiol., v. 21, no. 3, p. 218-221.

Gwirtz, K. H., J. V. Young, R. S. Byers, C. Alley, K. Levin, S. G. Walker, and R. K. Stoelting, 1999, The safety and efficacy of intrathecal opioid analgesia for acute postoperative pain: seven years' experience with 5969 surgical patients at Indiana University Hospital: Anesth.Analg., v. 88, no. 3, p. 599-604.

Haberal, M., R. Emiroglu, G. Arslan, E. Apek, H. Karakayali, and N. Bilgin, 2002, Living-donor nephrectomy under combined spinal-epidural anesthesia: Transplant.Proc., v. 34, no. 6, p. 2448-2449.

Hanaoka K. Experience in the use of Hanaoka's needles for spinal-continuous epidural anaesthesia (500 cases). 7th Asian Australian Congess of Anaesthesiologists Abstracts , 161-162. 1986.
Ref Type: Abstract

Harding, S. A., R. E. Collis, and B. M. Morgan, 1994, Meningitis after combined spinal-extradural anaesthesia in obstetrics: Br.J.Anaesth., v. 73, no. 4, p. 545-547.

Hayes, N. E., A. Aslani, and C. L. McCaul, 2011, Anaesthetic management of a patient with Liddle's syndrome for emergency caesarean hysterectomy: Int.J.Obstet.Anesth., v. 20, no. 2, p. 178-180.

Herbstman, C. H., J. B. Jaffee, K. J. Tuman, and L. M. Newman, 1998, An in vivo evaluation of four spinal needles used for the combined spinal-epidural technique: Anesth.Analg., v. 86, no. 3, p. 520-522.

Hirai, T., T. Kato, S. Kawabata, M. Enomoto, S. Tomizawa, T. Yoshii, K. Sakaki, K. Shinomiya, and A. Okawa, 2011, Adhesive Arachnoiditis with Extensive Syringomyelia and Giant Arachnoid Cyst Following Spinal and Epidural Anesthesia: A Case Report: Spine (Phila Pa 1976.).

Ho, K. M., W. D. Ngan Kee, and M. C. Poon, 1997, Combined spinal and epidural anesthesia in a parturient with idiopathic hypertrophic subaortic stenosis: Anesthesiology, v. 87, no. 1, p. 168-169.

Hoffmann, V. L., M. P. Vercauteren, P. W. Buczkowski, and G. L. Vanspringel, 1997, A new combined spinal-epidural apparatus: measurement of the distance to the epidural and subarachnoid spaces: Anaesthesia, v. 52, no. 4, p. 350-355.

Holmstrom, B., K. Laugaland, N. Rawal, and S. Hallberg, 1993, Combined spinal epidural block versus spinal and epidural block for orthopaedic surgery: Can.J.Anaesth., v. 40, no. 7, p. 601-606.

Holmstrom, B., N. Rawal, K. Axelsson, and P. A. Nydahl, 1995, Risk of catheter migration during combined spinal epidural block: percutaneous epiduroscopy study: Anesth.Analg., v. 80, no. 4, p. 747-753.

Horstman, D. J., E. T. Riley, and B. Carvalho, 2009, A randomized trial of maximum cephalad sensory blockade with single-shot spinal compared with combined spinal-epidural techniques for cesarean delivery: Anesth.Analg., v. 108, no. 1, p. 240-245.

Ithnin, F., Y. Lim, A. T. Sia, and C. E. Ocampo, 2006, Combined spinal epidural causes higher level of block than equivalent single-shot spinal anesthesia in elective cesarean patients: Anesth.Analg., v. 102, no. 2, p. 577-580.

Kasai, T., K. Yaegashi, M. Hirose, T. Fujita, and Y. Tanaka, 2003, Aseptic meningitis during combined continuous spinal and epidural analgesia: Acta Anaesthesiol.Scand., v. 47, no. 6, p. 775-776.

Katz, J., and H. Renck, 1987, Handbook of Thoraco-abdominal Nerve Block Hertfordshire, Prentice Hall PTR.

Kirsh, E. J., E. M. Worwag, M. Sinner, and G. W. Chodak, 2000, Using outcome data and patient satisfaction surveys to develop policies regarding minimum length of hospitalization after radical prostatectomy: Urology, v. 56, no. 1, p. 101-106.

Kodeih, M. G., A. A. Al-Alami, B. S. Atiyeh, and G. E. Kanazi, 2009, Combined spinal epidural anesthesia in an asthmatic patient undergoing abdominoplasty: Plast.Reconstr.Surg., v. 123, no. 3, p. 118e-120e.

Kopacz, D. J., and B. G. Bainton, 1996, Combined spinal epidural anesthesia: a new "hanging drop": Anesth.Analg., v. 82, no. 2, p. 433-434.

Kubina, P., A. Gupta, A. Oscarsson, K. Axelsson, and M. Bengtsson, 1997, Two cases of cauda equina syndrome following spinal-epidural anesthesia: Reg Anesth., v. 22, no. 5, p. 447-450.

Kucukguclu, S., H. Unlugenc, F. Gunenc, B. Kuvaki, N. Gokmen, S. Gunasti, S. Guclu, F. Yilmaz, and G. Isik, 2008, The influence of epidural volume extension on spinal block with hyperbaric or plain bupivacaine for Caesarean delivery: Eur.J.Anaesthesiol., v. 25, no. 4, p. 307-313.

Lew, E., S. W. Yeo, and E. Thomas, 2004, Combined spinal-epidural anesthesia using epidural volume extension leads to faster motor recovery after elective cesarean delivery: a prospective, randomized, double-blind study: Anesth.Analg., v. 98, no. 3, p. 810-814.

Lim, Y., W. Teoh, and A. T. Sia, 2006, Combined spinal epidural does not cause a higher sensory block than single shot spinal technique for cesarean delivery in laboring women: Anesth.Analg., v. 103, no. 6, p. 1540-1542.

Liu, S. S., and S. B. McDonald, 2001, Current issues in spinal anesthesia: Anesthesiology, v. 94, no. 5, p. 888-906.

Moiniche, S., J. B. Dahl, J. Rosenberg, and H. Kehlet, 1994, Colonic resection with early discharge after combined subarachnoid-epidural analgesia, preoperative glucocorticoids, and early postoperative mobilization and feeding in a pulmonary high-risk patient: Reg Anesth., v. 19, no. 5, p. 352-356.

Morton, G., and I. Bowler, 2001, Combined spinal-epidural as an alternative method of anaesthesia for a sigmoid-colectomy: Anaesthesia, v. 56, no. 8, p. 815-816.

Mumtaz, M. H., M. Daz, and M. Kuz, 1982, Another single space technique for orthopaedic surgery: Anaesthesia, v. 37, p. 90.

Ngan Kee, W. D., J. Shen, A. T. Chiu, I. Lok, and K. S. Khaw, 1999, Combined spinal-epidural analgesia in the management of labouring parturients with mitral stenosis: Anaesth.Intensive Care, v. 27, no. 5, p. 523-526.

Norris, M. C., S. T. Fogel, and C. Conway-Long, 2001, Combined spinal-epidural versus epidural labor analgesia: Anesthesiology, v. 95, no. 4, p. 913-920.

Paech, M. J., 1997, Unexplained neurologic deficit after uneventful combined spinal and epidural anesthesia for cesarean delivery: Reg Anesth., v. 22, no. 5, p. 479-482.

Puolakka, R., M. T. Pitkanen, and P. H. Rosenberg, 2001, Comparison of technical and block characteristics of different combined spinal and epidural anesthesia techniques: Reg Anesth.Pain Med., v. 26, no. 1, p. 17-23.

Rajakulendran, Y., S. Rahman, and N. Venkat, 1999, Long-term neurological complication following traumatic damage to the spinal cord with a 25 gauge whitacre spinal needle: Int.J.Obstet.Anesth., v. 8, no. 1, p. 62-66.

Rathmell, J. P., T. R. Lair, and B. Nauman, 2005, The role of intrathecal drugs in the treatment of acute pain: Anesth.Analg., v. 101, no. 5 Suppl, p. S30-S43.

Rawal, N., 2005, Combined spinal-epidural anaesthesia: Curr.Opin.Anaesthesiol., v. 18, no. 5, p. 518-521.

Rawal, N., B. Holmstrom, J. A. Crowhurst, and Z. A. Van, 2000, The combined spinal-epidural technique: Anesthesiol.Clin.North America., v. 18, no. 2, p. 267-295.

Rawal, N., J. Schollin, and G. Wesstrom, 1988, Epidural versus combined spinal epidural block for cesarean section: Acta Anaesthesiol.Scand., v. 32, no. 1, p. 61-66.

Rawal, N., Z. A. Van, B. Holmstrom, and J. A. Crowhurst, 1997, Combined spinal-epidural technique: Reg Anesth., v. 22, no. 5, p. 406-423.

Rosenberg, P. H., 1998, Novel technology: needles, microcatheters, and combined techniques: Reg Anesth.Pain Med., v. 23, no. 4, p. 363-369.

Sandkovsky, U., M. R. Mihu, A. Adeyeye, P. M. De Forest, and J. D. Nosanchuk, 2009, Iatrogenic meningitis in an obstetric patient after combined spinal-epidural analgesia: case report and review of the literature: South.Med.J., v. 102, no. 3, p. 287-290.

Schroter, J., D. D. Wa, V. Hoffmann, A. Bach, and J. Motsch, 1997, Epidural abscess after combined spinal-epidural block: Can.J.Anaesth., v. 44, no. 3, p. 300-304.

Shnaider, R., T. Ezri, P. Szmuk, S. Larson, R. D. Warters, and J. Katz, 2001, Combined spinal-epidural anesthesia for Cesarean section in a patient with peripartum dilated cardiomyopathy: Can.J.Anaesth., v. 48, no. 7, p. 681-683.

Simmons, S. W., A. M. Cyna, A. T. Dennis, and D. Hughes, 2007, Combined spinal-epidural versus epidural analgesia in labour: Cochrane.Database.Syst.Rev., no. 3, p. CD003401.

Somri, M. et al., 2011, The postoperative occurrence of cardio-respiratory adverse events in small infants undergoing gastrointestinal surgery: a prospective comparison of general anesthesia and combined spinal-epidural anesthesia: Pediatr.Surg.Int..

Somri, M., R. Tome, B. Yanovski, E. Asfandiarov, N. Carmi, J. Mogilner, B. David, and L. A. Gaitini, 2007, Combined spinal-epidural anesthesia in major abdominal surgery in high-risk neonates and infants: Paediatr.Anaesth., v. 17, no. 11, p. 1059-1065.

Soresi, A., 1937, Episubdural anesthesia: Anesthesia & Analgesia, v. 16, no. 1-6, p. 306-310.

Stamenkovic, D., V. Geric, M. Djordjevic, J. Raskovic, Z. Slavkovic, T. Randjelovic, and M. Karanikolas, 2009, Subarachnoid morphine, bupivacaine and fentanyl as part of combined spinal-epidural analgesia for low anterior resection. A prospective, randomised, double-blind clinical trial: Anaesth.Intensive Care, v. 37, no. 4, p. 552-560.

Stamenkovic, D. M., V. Geric, Z. Slavkovic, J. Raskovic, and M. Djordjevic, 2008, Combined spinal-epidural analgesia vs. intermittent bolus epidural analgesia for pain relief after major abdominal surgery. A prospective, randomised, double-blind clinical trial: Int.J.Clin.Pract., v. 62, no. 2, p. 255-262.

Stevens, D. S., and W. T. Edwards, 1999, Management of pain in intensive care settings: Surg.Clin.North Am., v. 79, no. 2, p. 371-386.

Stienstra, R., A. Dahan, B. Z. Alhadi, J. W. van Kleef, and A. G. Burm, 1996, Mechanism of action of an epidural top-up in combined spinal epidural anesthesia: Anesth.Analg., v. 83, no. 2, p. 382-386.

Stienstra, R., B. Z. Dilrosun-Alhadi, A. Dahan, J. W. van Kleef, B. T. Veering, and A. G. Burm, 1999, The epidural "top-up" in combined spinal-epidural anesthesia: the effect of volume versus dose: Anesth.Analg., v. 88, no. 4, p. 810-814.

Tahtaci, N., and M. Neyal, 2002, Combined spinal and epidural anaesthesia in elderly patients: Int.J.Clin.Pract., v. 56, no. 9, p. 655-658.

Turner, M. A., and N. A. Reifenberg, 1995, Combined spinal epidural anaesthesia: the single space double-barrel technique: Int.J.Obstet.Anesth., v. 4, no. 3, p. 158-160.

Tyagi, A., A. Kumar, A. K. Sethi, and M. Mohta, 2008, Epidural volume extension and intrathecal dose requirement: plain versus hyperbaric bupivacaine: Anesth.Analg., v. 107, no. 1, p. 333-338.

Urmey, W. F., 2000, Combined spinal epidural anesthesia: Techniques in regional anesthesia & pain management, v. 4, no. 1, p. 13-18.

Urmey, W. F., J. Stanton, M. Peterson, and N. E. Sharrock, 1995, Combined spinal-epidural anesthesia for outpatient surgery. Dose-response characteristics of intrathecal isobaric lidocaine using a 27-gauge Whitacre spinal needle: Anesthesiology, v. 83, no. 3, p. 528-534.

Urmey, W. F., J. Stanton, N. E. Sharrock, and E. Nigel, 1996, Combined Spinal/Epidural Anesthesia for Outpatient Surgery: Anesthesiology, v. 84, no. 2, p. 481-482.

van Zundert, A. A., G. Stultiens, J. J. Jakimowicz, D. Peek, W. G. van der Ham, H. H. Korsten, and J. A. Wildsmith, 2007, Laparoscopic cholecystectomy under segmental thoracic spinal anaesthesia: a feasibility study: Br.J.Anaesth., v. 98, no. 5, p. 682-686.

Van, d., V, N. Berends, B. Spitz, A. Teunkens, and E. Vandermeersch, 2004, Low-dose combined spinal-epidural anaesthesia vs. conventional epidural anaesthesia for Caesarean section in pre-eclampsia: a retrospective analysis: Eur.J.Anaesthesiol., v. 21, no. 6, p. 454-459.

Vasquez, C. E., R. R. Pereira, T. Tomita, A. Bedin, and R. A. Castro, 2002, [Meningitis after combined spinal-epidural analgesia for labor: case report]: Rev.Bras.Anestesiol., v. 52, no. 3, p. 330-334.

Vassiliev, D. V., E. U. Nystrom, and C. H. Leicht, 2001, Combined spinal and epidural anesthesia for labor and cesarean delivery in a patient with Guillain-Barre syndrome: Reg Anesth.Pain Med., v. 26, no. 2, p. 174-176.

Vercauteren, M. P., K. Geernaert, D. M. Vandeput, and H. Adriaensen, 1993, Combined continuous spinal-epidural anaesthesia with a single interspace, double-catheter technique: Anaesthesia, v. 48, no. 11, p. 1002-1004.

Waegerle, J. D., 1999, Combined spinal-epidural anesthesia/analgesia: CRNA., v. 10, no. 4, p. 155-164.

Wakamatsu, M., H. Katoh, U. Kondo, T. Yamamoto, and S. Tanaka, 1991, [Combined spinal and epidural anesthesia for orthopaedic surgery in the elderly]: Masui, v. 40, no. 12, p. 1766-1769.

Williams, R. K., W. J. McBride, and J. C. Abajian, 1997, Combined spinal and epidural anaesthesia for major abdominal surgery in infants: Can.J.Anaesth., v. 44, no. 5 Pt 1, p. 511-514.

9

Contraindications – Hemorrhage and Coagulopathy, and Patient Refusal

Bahanur Cekic[1] and Ahmet Besir[2]
[1]*Karadeniz Technical University School of the Medicine, Department of Anesthesiology and Critical Care,*
[2]*Trabzon Fatih Hospital, Department of Anesthesiology and Reanimation, Turkey*

1. Introduction

Widely used in surgical anesthesia, obstetric analgesia, -postoperative pain control and in the treatment of chronic pain, epidural techniques are contraindicated in such conditions as coagulopathy and other bleeding diathesis, patient refusal, hemodynamic instability, increased intracranial pressure and local or systemic infection.

Contraindications for epidural analgesia are patient reluctance, bleeding diathesis, hemodynamic instability, increased intracranial pressure and local or systemic infection. Contraindications are listed in Table 1.

Coagulation defects may be inherited or acquired (Table 2).

2. Contraindications - Hemorrhage and coagulopathy, and patient refusal

2.1 Coagulation and regulation of thrombin generation

Blood coagulation is a physiologic defense mechanism which develops as a response to a vascular damage and protects the integrity of the circulatory system. A hemostatic response to a trauma is a series of complex and interrelated events that necessitate interaction of the vessel wall, plasma proteins and platelets (Colman et al., 2001). This interaction results in one of the three outcomes: Hemorrhage, an appropriate hemostasis or a pathologic thrombosis (Hess & Lawson, 2006).

The cell-based coagulation method is frequently used today in understanding hemostasis. This model is divided into initiation, amplification and propagation phases (Hoffman & Monroe, 2001; Tanaka et al., 2009).

In the initiation phase, the surface of endothelium is activated by molecular or physical (traumatic or surgical) signals and it becomes the focal point of the procoagulant activity. The endogenous heparin molecule is removed from the surface of endothelium and the anticoagulant molecules become subject to thrombomoduline and antithrombin down regulation. A tissue factor is exposed to and the composition of endothelium surface phospholipids changes. To initiate formation of a clot, the tissue factor (TF) recruits coagulation zymogen factor VII. Activated factor VII (VIIa) converts factor IX and factor X into their active enzyme forms. Activated factor X(Xa) then converts prothrombin (fII) into thrombin (fIIa) and factor V (fV) into factor Va (fVa) (Adams et al., 2007). Thrombin so formed and fibrin which is formed from fibrinogen with the effect of thrombin are in very small amounts.

Coagulopathy and other bleeding diathesis
Patient refusal
Hemodynamic instability
Increased intracranial pressure
Local or systemic infection
Pre-existing neurological disorders

Table 1. Epidural blockage contraindications

Inherited
Hemophilia A and Hemophilia B
von Willebrand disease
Factor V deficiency
Inherited disorders of platelet disfunctions
Inherited hemorrhagic telangiectasia
Inherited thrombophilia
Acquired
Vitamin K deficiency
Drug-associated hemorrhage
Drug-associated hemorrhage
Disseminated intravascular coagulation
The Coagulopathy of Massive Trauma
Idiopathic thrombocytopenic purpura

Table 2. Classification of Coagulation Defects

In the amplification phase of thrombus, activated platelets bind to endothelium, activate factors V, XI and VIII and increase formation of thrombin through a positive feedback cycle (Adams et al., 2007; Hoffman & Monroe, 2001; Tanaka, 2009). Thrombocytes play a major role in localized clotting reactions in the trauma area. Thromobcytes bind and adhere to von Willebrand factor (vWF), thrombin, platelet receptors and subendothelial collagen in the trauma area and they form an aggregation. In this way, the surface for generation of required thrombin is formed for an effective hemostasis (Falati et al., 2002). As a result of the activation of platelets, cofactors Va and VIIIa quickly get localized on the surface of thrombocytes (Monroe et al., 1994). Factor Va accelerates and intensifies the activation of factor Xa. Factor VIIIa accelerates the binding of factor XIa to IXa (Adams et al., 2006) and enables continuation of procoagulant responses (Gailani & Broze, 1991).

In the propagation phase, fibrin polymerization and fibrin clotting occur. Thrombin first cleaves fibrinopeptide A and fibrinopeptide B particles from fibrinogen molecule and generates fibrin monomers and then fibrin polymers when these monomers aggregate. Thrombin also activates factor XIII to enable formation of cross-links among fibrin polymers and a firm fibrin clot (Hornyak & Shafer, 1992). A large amount of thrombin generated on the surface of thrombocyte is responsible for stabilization of the clot rather than supporting the polymerized fibrin (Hoffman & Monroe, 2007).

The coagulation cascade should be controlled and strictly monitored to confine it only in the area required. Many coagulation factors are serine protease and the coagulation process is regulated by serine protease inhibitors protein C and S, tissue factor pathway inhibitor (TFPI) and antithrombin. These agents inhibit clotting and formation of localized clot in the injured area. The fibrinolytic system in turn is activated and plays a role in dissolving the clot, healing the injury and reforming the tissue (Levy et al., 2010).

As a result, the competition of the procoagulant, anticoagulant, fibrinolytic and antifibrinolytic ways are regulated and remain in balance in human physiology. However, if a surgical stress, trauma or disease pushes any of these ways of competition out of balance, then it results in a pathologic condition that leads to either a hemorrhage or thrombosis (Hess & Lawson, 2006).

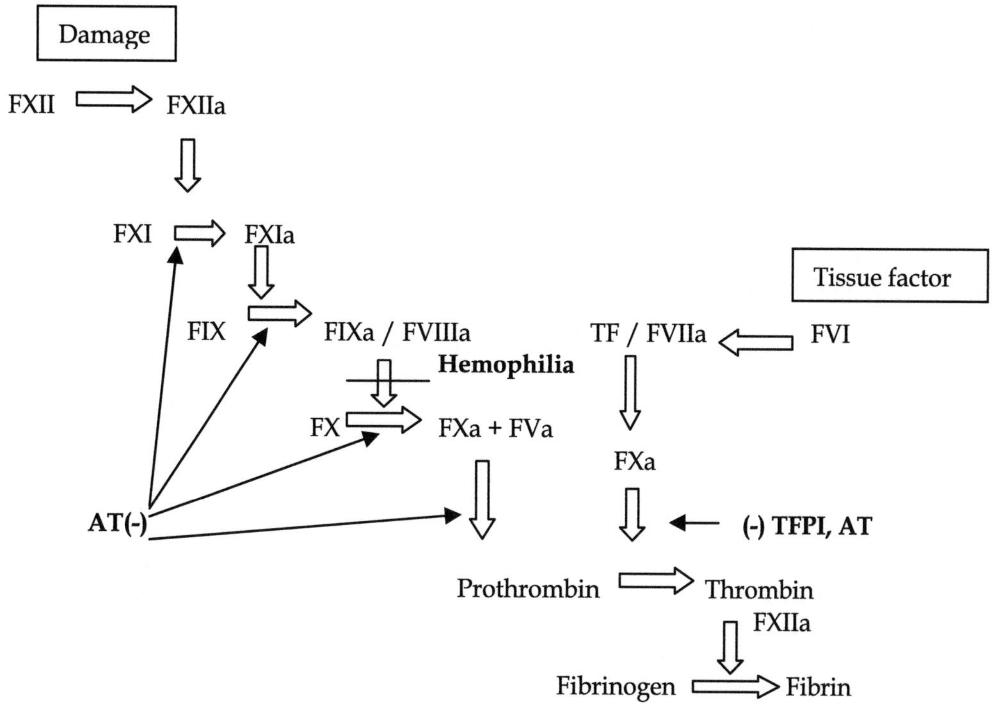

Fig. 1. Model of coagulation and regulation of thrombin generation.

2.2 Preoperative coagulation evaluation

The screening tests to determine bleeding risk in patients is ideally carried out in the preoperative period. Identification of hemostatic defects in this way helps in the preoperative period in the management of unpreventable bleeding. A history or a family history of bleeding in anamnesis increases the risk. The history of drug usage and the effect of used medicament to the coagulation cascade should be questioned.

Petechia, purpura, bleeding of nose or gums, hematuria, melena and other signs of bleeding should be noted as risk-increasing factors (Adams et al., 2007). Especially petechia (capillary) and purpura, which are physical characteristics of bleeding, as well as hematoma and ecchymose resulting from a large blood vessel bleeding should be well-explained. In detecting an inherited coagulopathy, presence of bleeding without any history of a disease or anticoagulant drug usage in the patient directly attracts the attention to an inherited defect.

Laboratory tests should be conducted in relation to the patient's clinical condition and history of bleeding and the type of planned surgery (Table 3).

Although preoperative scanning tests are not required in healthy individuals, neuraxial blockade, coagulation examinations and platelet counts should be conducted in cases in which clinical history indicates a probability of hemorrhage (Morgan et al., 2008).

Laboratory tests	Normal values
Prothrombin time	10-14 sec
Partial thromboplastin time	22-35 sec
International normalized ratio (INR)	0.80-1.30
Platelet Count	150.000-450.000/μL
Bleeding time	3-8 min
Thrombin time	9-25 sec
Fibrinogen assay	
Healthy individuals	200–400 mg/dL
With severe illness	400–800 mg/dL
Specific factors and inhibition levels	

Table 3. Laboratory tests and normal values

No testing is required in patients who have no history of bleeding and will undergo a minor surgery. In patients who have no history of bleeding but will undergo a major surgery, counts of partial thromboplastin time (PTT) and trombocyte is recommended. In patients with hemostatic disorders, the number of trombocytes, bleeding time, PTT and thromboplastin time should be measured (Adams et al., 2007).

Prothrombin time (PT) and activated partial thromboplastin time (aPTT) are the most widely used tests in screening coagulation disorders. PT is affected by reductions of Factors VII, X, V, and prothrombin such as occur with vitamin K antagonist therapy (Levy et al., 2008) or severe liver disease (Tripodi et al., 2007). aPTT is sensitive to gross reductions of Factors V, VIII, IX, XI, XII, and to a lesser extent, prothrombin (Tanaka et al., 2009). These screening coagulation tests are abnormal when there is a deficiency of one or more of the soluble coagulation factors (Hoffman & Monroe, 2007).

A consensus could not be reached about the minimum hemostatic condition required by regional techniques. One of the most common views is that if there is a thrombcyte function as a minimum threshold, then the hemostatic capacity is sufficient. Although a number of tests are carried out to assess the thrombocyte function today, it is not possible to arrive at definite information about the adequacy of coagulation. In these circumstances, the administration of a regional anesthesia and the minimum hemostatic condition that is required to apply the anesthesia can be realized if;

- the number of functional platelets >80-100 000 μL^{-1},
- international normalized ratio (INR) < 1.5,
- activated prothrombin time (aPTT) <45 sec.

(Llau et al., 2005; Tyagi & Bhattacharya, 2002; Mentegazziet al., 2005).

2.3 Coagulation defects

2.3.1 Inherited coagulation defects

Inherited coagulation defects generally appear because of the absence or insufficiency of a single coagulation factor.

2.3.1.1 Hemophilia A and hemophilia B

Hemophilia A and B are X-linked recessively inherited disorders. The incidence of hemophilia is 1 in 5000 male births an that of hemophilia B is 1 in 30000 (Tuddenham & Cooper, 1994).

Characterized by excessive bleeding in various parts of the body, hemophilia develops due to a mutation of factor VIII (Hemophilia A) and factor IX (Hemophilia B) coagulation genes. The chance of inheriting a gene defect from a hemophilia carrier is 50%. A patient's son is affected with a chance of 50% at every pregnancy and her daughter, who is also a carrier of the disease, is also affected with a chance of 50% (Cahill & Colvin, 1997). However, hemophilia may also develop in 30% of the cases as a result of a spontaneous mutation without any history of hemophilia in the family (Mannucci & Tuddenham, 2001).

Hemophilia is classified according to the level of the clotting factor. A hundred percent of the said factor which is contained in 1 mL of normal plasma is referred to as 1 unit. Normal plasma activity is between 5 $U.dl^{-1}$ and 15 $U.dl^{-1}$ (50-150%) (DiMichele & Neufeld, 1998). The level of normal factor in seriously affected patients is <1%, in moderately affected 1-4% and in mildly affected 5-50% (Cahill & Colvin, 1997). While those with serious hemophilia are susceptible to spontaneous bleeding episodes, the ones with mild hemophilia have bleeding after a trauma or surgery (Mannucci & Tuddenham, 2001).

There are case reports in the literature notifying the occurrence of an epidural hematoma following a lumbar puncture in patients who were not known to have hemophilia (Bernhardt et al., 2008; Faillace et al., 1989). The use of a regional block in patients with bleeding disorders is controversial because of the risk of developing hematoma which leads to epidural or spinal bleeding and a permanent neurological damage. However, the use of a regional block is not contraindicated when the coagulation tests (platelet quantity, PT, aPTT, INR and fibrinogen) are normal and the relevant factor level is >50$IU.dl^{-1}$ or is raised to >50$IU.dl^{-1}$ through a prophylactic treatment (Lee et al., 2006; Silverman et al., 1993; , Dhar et al., 2003).

An epidural intervention should be applied with a midline approach by an experienced anesthetist (Abramovitz & Beilin, 2003). A mixture of low-dose local anesthetics and narcotics should be used to attain analgesia by protecting the motor function (Dhar et al., 2003). Motor block measurements should be carried out frequently until the catheter is removed. If the degree of the motor block is higher than expected and the length of anesthesia is prolonged, a magnetic resonance imaging should be made to control development of an epidural hematoma.

It is important to check the factor levels before the epidural catheter is removed.

2.3.1.2 von Willebrand disease (vWD)

Von Willebrand disease (vWD) is an inherited hematologic disorder which involves vWF deficiency and is the most prevailing bleeding disorder affecting nearly 1% of the general population (Rodeghiero et al., 1987). vWD is divided into three types according to the qualitative and quantitative deficiency of the vWF level. The vWF level is decreased in vWD Type 1; it is normal in Type 2, but there is a function disorder. The vWF deficiency is serious in vWD Type 3. The most common one is Type 1 which constitutes approximately 70% of the cases. While vWD Types 1 and 2 are inherited autosomal dominantly, Type 3 is inherited autosomal recessively (Lee et al., 2006).

vWF is necessary for adhesion of platelets to form a platelet clump in an injured endothelium. It is also the carrier protein of Factor VIII. When vWF is deficient, the time of bleeding is prolonged and patients generally have abnormal bleedings such as epistaxis, menorrhagia and postpartum bleeding (Varughese &Cohen, 2007). Tendency to bleeding is moderate in vWD Type 1 and 2, but serious in Type 3. Pregnant women with vWD have a progressively increasing FVIII coagulation activity (FVIII:C), and vWF antigen (vWF:Ag) and vWF activity (vWF:AC) during pregnancy, which all return to the baseline after delivery (Greer et al., 1991; Punnonen et al., 1981; Kadir et al., 1998). The increase in the variables showing such platelet activity is apparent in pregnant women with vWD Type 1, moderate in Type 2 and very little or nil in Type 3. Because of the differences in hemostatic responses, the factor levels with plasma vWF:Ag, VWF:AC and FVIII:C should regularly be monitored in pregnant women with vWD.

When the vWF activity becomes <50 IU.dl^{-1} during an invasive intervention or a delivery, a prophylactic treatment should be initiated using a coagulation factor concentrate with vWF. A prophylactic treatment is not necessary at delivery in women with vWD Type 1. Treatment becomes necessary in vWD Type 2 if a cesarean section is being carried out or a perineal trauma occurred. Women with vWD Type 3 require treatment in all types of delivery (Lee et al., 2006).

The risk of developing a spinal hematoma after an epidural anesthesia is very rare in obstetric patients (1:200000). However, this risk increases in patients with serious coagulopathy (Moen et al., 2004). Neuraxial interventions are contraindicated in patients with vWD whose bleeding disorders are not healed. Although vWD is quite common among bleeding disorders, there are very few case reports describing an anesthetic method for vWD patients (Hara et at., 2009; Caliezi et al., 1998; Jones et al., 1999; Milaskiewicz et al., 1990; Cohen et al., 1989). Paucity of large case series showing that epidural interventions are safe makes anesthetists hesitate when conducting anesthesia on women with vWD.

When the vWF activity becomes >50 IU.dl^{-1} in women with vWD Type 1 or this value is reached through replacement, an epidural anesthesia can safely be administered. However, the decision of using an epidural anesthesia should be made jointly by an experienced anesthetist, a hematologist and a gynecologist (Lee et al., 2006). Epidural anesthesia is not recommended for patients with vWD Type 2 and 3 (Pasi et al., 2004). An epidural anesthesia should be administered by an experienced anesthetist.

2.3.1.3 Factor V deficiency

Factor V deficiency is a congenital bleeding disorder which prevails very rarely (1 in 1000000) in the population (Asselta et al., 2006). Factor V itinerates as an inactive cofactor in the plasma and is activated by thrombin. Activated factor V works as a cofactor with factor VIIIa and factor Xa to convert prothrombin into thrombin (Fogerty & Connors, 2009).

Factor V deficiency is classified as quantitative (type 1) and qualitative (type II) (Asselta et al., 2006). When the plasma FV antigen level becomes <15%, it is classified as a serious Type I deficiency and when it becomes <60-65%, as a moderate Type I deficiency. A moderate to serious level of bleeding occurs in serious Type I deficiency (Asselta et al., 2006; Vellinga et al., 2006).

There is no evident information on the use of neuraxial techniques in these patients. However, it was reported that the neuraxial techniques were safe in labor epidural analgesia when the FV level becomes > 60% (Le Gouez et al., 2011). In pregnancy, prothrombin time (PT) can be normal although the FV level is low (Cerneca et al., 1997). For this reason, PT alone is not sufficient in determining the FV level. The FV level should be reassessed to be able to remove the epidural catheter safely (Kadir et al., 2009).

2.3.1.4 Inherited hemorrhagic telangiectasia

Hereditary hemorrhagic telangiectasia (HHT), also known as the Osler-Weber-Rendu Syndrome, is a congenital autosomal dominant multiple vascular dysplasia which is seen in 1 person out of 5000-8000 (Begbie et al., 2003). This disease is characterized by multiple arteriovenous malformations (AVMs) associated with the lack of capillaries joining arteries with veins in the solid organs of a body and telangiectasis of cutaneous and mucous membranes (Hereditary Hemorrhagic Telangiectasia Foundation International Inc., 2007). Vascular dysplasia is mostly seen in pulmonary, cerebral, gastrointestinal and spinal vascular structures. The course of the disease may progress silently or in a life-threatening manner from a high-output heart failure secondary to arteriovenous shunting, a systemic emboli, rupture of AVMs up to a fatal hemorrhage (Lomax & Edgcombe, 2009).

A successful anesthesia can be administered to patients with HHT only if the existing specific AVMs are known, cardiovascular instability is avoided and a prophylaxis is applied for systemic emboli that may develop as a result of AVM shunting. Spinal AVMs constitute a relative contraindication for regional techniques (Lomax & Edgcombe, 2009).

2.3.1.5 Inherited disorders of platelet dysfunctions

2.3.1.5.1 Glanzmann's thrombasthenia

Glanzmann's Thrombasthenia a congenital, hereditary and hemorrhagic disorder caused by qualitative and quantitative impairment of platelet glycoprotein (GP) IIb/IIIa. Bleeding such as purpura, epistaxis, gingival hemorrhage and menorrhagia are seen in these patients due to defective platelets in the formation of hemostatic clump. The disorder can clinically be diagnosed through the signs of normal number of platelets, abnormal platelet aggregation and prolonged bleeding time (George et al., 1990).

2.3.1.5.2 Bernard-Soulier syndrome

Bernard-Soulier syndrome is a rarely seen bleeding disorder inherited in an autosomal recessive way. This disease develops in connection with the abnormality or lack of platelet membrane glycoprotein GPIb-V-IX and it is characterized by giant platelets, thrombocytopenia in various grades and prolonged bleeding time (Kostopanagiotou et al., 2004). Clinically it progresses with excessive bleeding not proportionate to the degree of thrombocytopenia and the bleedings are fatal (Bernard, 1983).

2.3.1.6 Inherited thrombophilia

2.3.1.6.1 Protein C deficiency

Protein C deficiency is a thrombotic disease inherited in an autosomal dominant way with a prevalence of 0.2-0.5% in the population (Aiach et al., 1997; Reitsma, 1997; Walker, 1997). Protein C is the central protein of the major antithrombotic system of hemostasis. Protein C itinerates in the plasma as an inactive zymogen linked to vitamin K. It is activated in endothelium by the thrombomodulin-thrombin complex. Activated Protein C inactivates coagulation factor Va and VIIIa. It also has a fibrinolysis function by neutralizing inhibitor of tissue-type plasminogen activator (TPAI) (Esmon, 1989).

Protein C deficiency is at increased risk for deep vein thrombosis and pulmonary embolism, especially during pregnancy and the post partum period. For this reason patients are administered thromboemboli propylaxis and thrombosis therapy during preoperative and postoperative periods. Continuation of anticoagulation therapy, on the other hand, may increase the risk of re-bleeding with life-threatening mass effect (Ranasinghe et al., 2008; Sternberg et al., 1991). It is important to discuss a benefit-loss balance for these patients before a neuraxial procedure.

2.3.1.6.2 Antithrombin III deficiency

Antithrombin III deficiency is a hereditary disorder received in an autosomal dominant way and is seen in the population at a rate between 1/2000 and 1/5000 (Rosenberg, 1975). It is a glycoprotein which inhibits factor IIa (thrombin) and antithrombin factor Xa. Antithrombin deficiency is of the highest clinical significance among the congenital thrombophilia as it causes life-threatening thromboses (Maclean & Tait, 2007). A long-lasting anticoagulant therapy becomes inevitable in these patients due to a recurring venous thromboemboli (VTE) risk. A prophylactic anticoagulation should be administered to asymptomatic individuals especially in high-risk episodes (e.g. surgery, immobility and pregnancy) (Birnbach & Grunebaum, 1991).

LMWH is particularly recommended as an anticoagulant treatment of antithrombin deficiency. The use of LMWH is restricted in regional anesthesia due to the risk of bleeding. The American Society of Regional Anesthesia (ASRA) guidelines today recommends to discontinue the treatment at least 24 h before any neuraxial procedure is initiated (if the treatment is used in the right intensity) (Horlocker et al., 2003). This period of discontinued anticoagulant treatment in patients with high risk of VTE constitute a critical interval. In the last ten years, the use of antithrombin concentrations is recommended in high-risk situations (e.g. cesarean section, elective surgery and delivery) (Tiede et al., 2008). There are a limited number of case reports stating successful administration of epidural anesthesia and analgesia under an antithrombin treatment in hereditary antithrombin deficiency (Pamnani et al., 2010).

2.3.2 Acquired coagulation defects

2.3.2.1 Vitamin K deficiency

Patients with vitamin K deficiency should be given oral or parenteral treatment depending on the reason of the deficiency. In a vitamin K deficiency, only the prothrombin time (PTT) is prolonged. Vitamin K deficiency is extremely common among hospitalized patients for multiple reasons. Poor diet (lack of leafy vegetables) often results in hospitalization.

Warfarin is a competitive inhibitor of vitamin K. The amount of vitamin K required to reverse its effect depends on the amount of warfarin in blood.

2.3.2.2 Drug-associated hemorrhage

Drug-associated hemorrhage may stem from heparin, vitamin K antagonists, platelet aggregation inhibitors, glycoprotein IIb/IIIa inhibitors or direct thrombin inhibitors.

Regional anesthesia in the presence of anticoagulation

a. Anesthetists should be aware of the potential risk of bleeding when conducting regional anesthesia techniques in patients who receive antithrombotic treatment and are planned to undergo a surgery. When a potent antithrombotic drug was involved, this often has resulted in avoidance of regional anesthesia techniques due to the concern about the patient's safety. Therefore, some national anesthesia societies have published guidelines describing how to safely conduct regional anesthesia when using antiplatelet, anticoagulant and thrombolytic medication. The first national recommendations on neuraxial anesthesia and antithrombotic drugs were published by the German Society for Anesthesiology and Intensive Care in 1997 (Gogarten et al., 1997), followed by the American Society of Regional Anesthesia (ASRA) in 1998 (Horlocker & Wedel, 1998), and Belgian anesthesiologists in 2000 (Belgian Guidelines 2000). In this context, there are a large number of recommendations approved by scientific anesthesia societies (Horlocker et al., 2003; Llau et al., 2005; Vandermeulen et al., 2005; Samama et al., 2002). This enabled comparison of similarities and differences in some important situations (Llau et al., 2007).

The European Society of Anesthesiology (ESA) has recently published recommendations about the time intervals between the neuraxial blockage and removal of the catheter and the administration of an anticoagulant when anticoagulant agents are being used (Gogarten et al., 2010). Such guidelines are continuously being updated because new anticoagulants are regularly being developed and they are based on large case series, case reports and pharmacologic data of anticoagulant drugs rather than controlled studies.

Administrators of neuraxial block on patients receiving antithrombotic treatment should be weary of possible hematoma formation resulting into neurologic deficit. Epidural hematoma related to neuraxial anesthesia is a rare but potentially devastating complication (Guffey et al., 2010; Li et al., 2010; Han et al., 2010). The risk of hemorrhage is lowest in spinal anesthesia, which employs fine needles, and highest in epidural catheter anesthesia, which requires the largest needle gauges available. Nearly half of all cases of bleeding occur during the removal of an epidural catheter, and this procedure must be regarded as critical as catheter insertion

(Vandermeulen et al., 1994). Catheter manipulation and removal carry similar risks to insertion, and the same criteria should apply. Appropriate neurological monitoring is essential during the postoperative recovery period and following catheter removal.

b. Antithrombotic drugs and Regional Anesthesia

This is used if it is believed to be more beneficial than the alternative methods. Anticoagulants, antiplatelet drugs and thrombolytics are used for the prevention and treatment of stroke, myocardial infarction, deep vein thrombosis, and pulmonary embolism in many patients undergoing surgery (Table 4). (Donegan et al., 2007). The risk of developing epidural hematoma is reduced if care is taken for the characteristics of these drugs and the safe time intervals needed for administering the regional technique (Llau et al., 2001). Neuraxial anesthesia can be accepted in these patients only if coagulation is optimized and monitoring is done during the application.

Drugs groups
Heparins
Anti- Xa agents
Direct thrombin inhibitors
Vit K Antagonists
Antiplatelet drugs

Table 4. Antithrombotic drugs

Regional anesthesia in patients on treatment with unfractionated heparins

Factor IIa produces an anticoagulant effect by inhibiting the antithrombin III enzyme activity on IXa and Xa (Weitz, 1997; Hirsh & Raschke, 2004). Unfractional heparin (UH) is administered subcutaneously (sc) or intravenously (iv). Its half-life varies according to the dose (Llau et al., 2007).

Coagulation tests need not be done for patients who receive sc UH in prophylactic doses (<15000IU/day) However, a thrombocyte count should be carried out in patients who have received treatment for more than 5 days and for whom there is a need to distinguish heparin-induced thrombocytopenia. The treatment should be suspended 2 to 4h before removing the catheter. The next heparin dose should be postponed until 1h after the procedure (Gogarten et al., 2010).

Although the UH dose used in venous thromboprophylaxis is safe, the risk of bleeding increases in therapeutic doses. For this reason, insertion and removal of catheters is contraindicating in patients receiving therapeutic treatment. If a safe removal of neuraxial blockage or catheter is planned, administration of intravenous (iv) heparin should be suspended for at least 4h and it should be ascertained before the procedure that aPTT, activated clotting time (ACT), anti-Xa activity and thrombocyte quantity are all normal. It should be avoided for 2h in low doses if an intraoperative heparinization is planned and for 6-12 hours if a full heparinization is planned (Gogarten et al., 2010).

Regional anesthesia in patients on treatment with low molecular weight heparins

This is widely used to prevent and treat deep vein thrombosis (DVT) by inhibiting factor Xa formation. It became superior to the other anticoagulants as it has high level of bioavailability, the risk of bleeding is low and it can easily be used without any need for monitoring blood clotting (Vandermeulen, 2010). LMWH reaches the peak plasma level approximately 4h after a subcutaneous procedure and its activity continues for 24h (Hirsh et al., 2001).

In order to avoid any bleeding complication, there must be at least 12h (in prophylactic dose of LMWH) or 24h (in therapeutic dose of LMWH) between the last dose of LMWH and the removal of the neuraxial blockage or epidural catheter (Vandermeulen et al., 1994; Bergqvist et al., 1993). The next LMWH dose should be applied 4h after the epidural/spinal puncture or catheter removal (Gogarten et al., 2010). The probability of developing a heparin-induced thrombocytopenia (HIT) after LMWH is ten times less as compared to UH (Warkentin et al., 1995).

However, a thrombocyte count is recommended after using LMWH for more than 5 days (Vandermeulen, 2010).

Danaparoid

Danaparoid is a glycosaminoglycan containing 84% heparan sulphate, 12% dermatan sulphate and 4% chondroitin sulphate. Its anti-thrombotic effect occurs through antithrombin-induced inhibition of factor Xa (Ibbotson & Perry, 2002). Coagulation is monitored by using only the anti-X activity. It is used as an alternative to UH and LMWH in prevention and treatment of pulmonary emboli and VTE in patients with a history of danaparoid HIT (Wilde & Markham, 1997). Since it has a 22-hour elimination half-life, a preoperative danaparoid administration should be avoided in patients who are planned to undergo a neuraxial blockage (Gogarten et al., 2010).

Regional anesthesia in patients on treatment with factor Xa inhibitors

Fondaparinux

Fondaparinux is a selective reversible inhibitor of coagulation factor Xa. It has a high affinity with antithrombin III without affecting active thrombin and platelet aggregation (Weitz et al., 2004).

A single dose of it is used daily because the half-life of this compound is 18-21h (Boneu et al., 1995). The safe interval between a fondaparinux application and a single-shot neuraxial anesthesia is 6h. The catheter can be removed 36h after the last dose. A Fondaparinux dose should be given at least 12 hours after removing the catheter (Llau Pitarch et al., 2005).

Rivaroxaban

Rivaroxaban is a selective factor Xa inhibitor. It is currently administered orally as a single dose of 10 mg to prevent a deep vein thrombosis following a total hip and knee prosthesis surgery. It reaches a maximum plasma level in 2-4h. APTT is prolonged depending on the dose. It prolongs PT with a close correlation with the plasma concentration (Kubitza et al., 2005). A time interval of 22-26h is required between the last dose of rivaroxaban and removal of the neuraxial catheter (Gogarten et al., 2010). The next dose of rivaroxaban should be applied 4-6 h after the catheter is removed (Gogarten et al., 2010).

Apixaban

Apixaban is an oral, reversible, rivaroxaban-linked direct inhibitor of factor Xa. Its half-life is between 10-15 h (Weitz et al., 2008). There must be a time interval of 26-30h between the last dose of apixaban (2.5mg) and catheter removal. Its next dose should be given 4-6 hours after catheter removal (Gogarten et al., 2010).

Regional anesthesia in patients treated with direct thrombin inhibitors

This group of drugs uses direct selective thrombin inhibition to produce both perioperative thromboprophylaxis and therapeutic anticoagulation. They also inactivate thrombin-linked fibrin and prevent thrombus from further growing (Gogarten et al., 2010). Their anticoagulant effects can be monitored using aPTT and ecarin clotting time (ECT) (Greinacher, 2004).

Hirudins: bivalirudin, desirudin and lepirudin

All hirudins are potent anticoagulants and bind thrombin irreversibly. They can be used in HIT patients because they do not interact with thrombocyte factors (Lubenow & Greinacher, 2002). Lepirudin and desirudin have a half-life of 1.3-2 h and bivalirudin 25-30 min (Robson et al., 2002; Dasgupta et al., 2000). In patients with normal renal function, there must be at least 8-10 h of time between the last dose of a hirudin and insertion of a neuraxial blockage / catheter or removal of the catheter. The next dose may be given 2-4 h after catheter removal.

Argatroban

Argatroban is a reversible direct thrombin inhibitor (Kaplan, 2003; Kathiresan et al., 2002). Its half-life is 35-45 min (Yeh & Jang, 2006). It is applied intravenously 0.5-2 μkg/min in patients with normal organ functions and it prolongs aPTT about 1.5 to 3 times that of the normal. There must be at least 4 h of time between the last dose of argatroban and insertion or removal of a neuraxial blockage / catheter. The next dose may be given 2 h after catheter removal.

Dabigatran

Dabigatran oral is a reversible thrombin inhibitor which is used for VTE prophylaxis (Weitz et al., 2008). It is used every other day because it has a long half-life (12-17 h). The first dose of dabigatran is applied 4 h postoperatively. There must be 4 h between its last dose and catheter removal. The next dabigatran dose can be given 2 h after catheter removal (Boehringer-Ingelheim, 2009).

Regional anesthesia in patients treated with Vit K Antagonists

Neuraxial block is definitely contraindicated in patients treated with Vit K antagonists such as acenocoumarol, phenprocoumon and warfarin. All of these drugs cause coagulation factor II, VII, IX and X deficiencies and protein C and S inhibitions (Ansell et al., 2004). A few days after discontinuation of these drugs, coagulation returns to normal; the progress can be controlled by using the international normalized ratio (INR). Vit K antagonists are discontinued 3-5 days prior to the administration of regional technique in the preoperative period and one of the other anticoagulants, particularly LMWH, is temporarily administered to the patient (Dunn & Turpie 2003). INR should be <1.4 before the regional technique. If the epidural catheter needs to be removed under a warfarin therapy, it should be removed before the anticoagulant effect begins (INR<1.4) (Llau Pitarch et al., 2005).

Regional anesthesia in patients on treatment with antiplatelet drugs

Antiplatelet agents are compounds used for preventing arterial thrombosis in various clinical processes (Samama et al., 2002; Tufano et al., 2002). They inhibit platelet functions and are classified according to their mechanisms of action:

Acetylsalicylic acid (ASA)

ASA shows its effect by irreversibly inhibiting the cyclooxygenase enzyme. Its time of action is as long as a platelet life (7-10 days) (Vandermeulen, 2010). The bleeding effect of ASA depends on its dose (Serebruany et al., 2005). It inhibits generation of thromboxane A_2 in low doses and prostacyclin in high doses. It was shown that the risk of spontaneous bleeding was quite low in patients having normal quantity of platelets who use low doses of ASA during an anti platelet treatment (McQuaid & Laine, 2006). When ASA or non-steroidal anti-inflammatory drugs (NSAIDS) are used alone, the risk of a spinal/epidural hematoma does not increase and they do not constitute a contraindication in using regional techniques. A limited number of studies in the literature demonstrate that spinal hematoma does not pose and extra risk in this group of patients CLASP (Collaborative Low-dose Aspirin Study in Pregnancy) (Collaborative Group., 1994; Horlocker et al., 1995; Horlocker et al., 2002).

It was shown that a postoperative thromboprophylaxis was more beneficial than a preoperative one (Hull et al., 2000).

For this reason, it is recommended to administer a VTE prophylaxis involving ASA in the postoperative period following the regional technique (Llau et al., 2005).

The suggestion that the use of ASA should be discontinued 7 days before the operation in patients getting ready for an operation is outstanding among other recommendations (Kövesi & Royston, 2002). Having a break for 7 days will increase the risk of developing cardiovascular and neurologic complication (Burger et al., 2005). It is recommended that antiaggregants, ASA in particular, should be restarted between postoperative 6 and 24 h (Llau et al., 2007).

Thienopyridines

Thienopyridines which consist of ticlopidine and clopidogrel show their effect by antagonizing adenosine diphosphate (ADP) in the purine receptors of thrombocytes. These drugs reach their peek activity 3-5 days after having been received and their antiaggregant effect extents up to 7-10 days (Patrono et al., 2004). The half-life of ticlopidine is 30-50 h and that of clopidogrel is 120 h (Vandermeulen, 2010). Thienopyridines have a very large antiaggregant capacity. There is no data indicating that they are being safely used in regional techniques. However, there are reports notifying development of a spinal epidural hematoma following the neuraxial block in a clopidogrel therapy (Litz et al., 2004). Today, it is not recommended to administer a regional technique to patients who are under the influence of ticlopidine or clopidogrel. Nevertheless, a regional technique can safely be administered after suspending the clopidogrel therapy for 7 days and the ticlopidine therapy for 10 days (Llau et al., 2007).

GP IIb/IIIa receptor antagonists

GPIIb/IIIa receptor antagonists which consist of abciximab, tirofiban and eptifibatide are among the most effective drugs today for inhibition of platelet aggregation. They show their effect by reversibly inhibiting glycoprotein IIb/IIIa receptors of platelets. They are mostly used in treating acute coronary syndrome. After being applied, eptifibatide/tirofiban is effective for 8-10 h and abciximab for 24-48. A thrombocytopenia may develop within 1 to 24 hours after they are administered (Dasgupta et al., 2000; Huang & Hong, 2004). Use of a regional technique or removal of catheter can be done 8 h after the last dose of eptifibatide/tirofiban or 24-48 h after the last dose of abciximab (Gogarten, 2006). A thrombocyte count should however be done to confirm that there is no thrombocytopenia (Llau et al., 2007). Safe time interval before and after a neuraxial block in patients receiving antithrombotic drugs were defined in table 5.

	Route of administered	before NB/CW	after NB/CW
Unfractionated heparin	sc, iv	4h	1h
Low-molecular-weight heparins			
prophylactic	sc	12h	4h
therapeutic	sc	24h	4h
Danaparoid	sc	CI	CI
Factor Xa inhibitors			
Fondaparinux	sc	36-42h	6-12h
Rivaroxaban	oral	22-26h	4-6h
Apixaban	oral	26-30h	4-6h
Direct thrombin inhibitors			
Hirudins	sc, iv	8-10h	2-4h
Argatroban	iv	4h	2h
Dabigatran	oral	4h	2h
Vit K Antagonists			
warfarin	oral	INR<1.4	Restart after CW
Antiplatelet drugs			
Acetylsalicylic acid (ASA) *	oral	No CI	Postoperative 6-24h
Thienopyridines			
Ticlopidine	oral	10 days	-
Clopidogrel	oral	7 days	-
GP IIb/IIIa receptor antagonists			
Abciximab	iv	24-48 h	-
Eptifibatide or tirofiban	iv	8 h	-

NB:Neuraxial block;CW:Catheter withdrawalCI:Contraindication INR:International normalized ratio
* When ASA is given as a single drug, neuraxial block could be performed freely

Table 5. Safe time interval before and after a neuraxial block in patients receiving antithrombotic drugs

2.3.2.3 Disseminated intravascular coagulation (DIC)

The magnitude of a trauma may be accompanied by a coagulation change. Specific injuries such as impairment of the central nervous system, bone fractures and amniotic fluid emboli are often accompanied by disseminated intravascular coagulation (DIC) (Levi & Ten, 1993). The embolized material gains strength with thromboplastin and causes intravascular coagulation as the direct clotting factors are consumed (Hess & Lawson, 2006).

In patients with DIC following an acute trauma, the level of fibrinogen usually goes down first. This drop in fibrinogen is followed by consumption of other coagulation factors. The prothrombin time (PTT) and the active partial thromboplastin time (aPTT) are prolonged and the number of platelets and the level of fibrinogen drop (Gando et al., 1992; Ordog et al., 1985).

In patients with post-traumatic DIC, a distinct drop in the levels of protein C and antithrombin indicates an anticoagulant activity deficiency (Gando, 2001; Gando et al.,1988; Gando et al., 1992; Chesebroet al., 2009).

DIC divides into two phenomena, fibrinolitic (hemorrhagic) and antifibrinolitic (thrombotic). DIC has the character of a fibrinolitic phenomenon in the early stage of the trauma, that is, after approximately 24-48 h and is accompanied by massive hemorrhages (Sawamura et al., 2009). DIC becomes a thrombotic phenomenon in the later stage of the trauma, that is, after approximately 3-5 days. It is then characterized by a development of multiorgan dysfunction (MODS) (Gando, 2001).

2.3.2.4 The coagulopathy of massive trauma

In patients with serious trauma, coagulopathy is associated with the loss, consumption and dysfunction of coagulation factors. Coagulopathy is aggravated by hemodilution, acidosis and hypothermia (Armand & Hess, 2003).

Hemodilution occurs due to a massive blood loss. A massive bleeding causes a decrease in the number of platelets, shortening of coagulation time, an increase in fibrinogen turnover and consumption of coagulation factors (Turpini & Stefanini, 1959). Moreover, the liquid and blood products and massive transfusion of hypovolemia result in a dilution which intensifies the coagulopathy (Armand & Hess, 2003).

Acidosis occurs as a result of tissue hypoperfusion and hypoxia associated with a shock. When pH becomes <7.1, the propagation stage of thrombosis comes to be blocked (Martini, 2009).

A serious hypothermia decreases coagulation enzyme activity and impairs platelet functions (Martini, 2009; Wolberg et al., 2004).

2.3.2.5 Idiopathic thrombocytopenic purpura (ITP)

Idiopathic thrombocytopenic purpura (ITP) is an autoimmune thrombocytopenic coagulopathy, which is seen in 1 person out of 100000. It is characterized by a persistent thrombocytopenia which develops as a result of destruction of platelets by the reticuloendothelial system due to antibodies that adhere to thrombocytes (Kessler et al., 1982). Platelets have an important role in continuation of coagulation cascade in the hemostatic system and in formation of hemostatic clumps (Beilin et al., 1997). A low number of platelets impairs surgical hemostasis by increasing the risk of hemorrhage and may cause anesthetic complications such as hematoma (Chow et al., 2011). Patients with ITP should be distinguished from the other causes of thrombocytopenia including sepsis, pregnancy-induced hypertension, disseminated intravascular coagulation, drug-induced thrombocytopenia, thrombocytopenia associated with autoimmune diseases (systemic lupus erythematosus, thrombotic thrombocytopenic purpura, hemolytic uremic syndrome, and hereditary forms of thrombocytopenia) (Webert et al., 2003).

The number of platelets helps distinguish the other diseases involving coagulopathy in clinical settings.

In patients with ITP, platelet functions are normal, and the number of platelets is low and stable (Abramovitz &Beilin,2003).

In assessing platelet functions of ITP patients, the bedside tests of bleeding time and thromboelastography as well as platelet function analysis tests (aggregometry or flow cytometry) can be used (Beilin et al., 1997).

Traditionally, regional anesthesia is believed to be contraindicating in thrombocytopenia. What lies behind this belief is that the absolute cut-off point of platelets was accepted to be 100.000/mm^{-3} because the bleeding time was prolonged when the number of platelets went below 100.000/mm^{-3}. Following the belief that a neuraxial anesthesia is not safe below the absolute platelet number, many clinicians avoid carrying out any epidural procedures (Harker & Slichter, 1972; Bromage, 1993). Many textbooks and articles of our time suggest that epidural applications can be done safely at <100.000/mm^{-3} (Beilin et al., 1997; Rasmus et al., 1989; Rolbin et al., 1988; British Committee for Standards in Haematology General Haematology Task Force, 2003). Most of the anesthetists believe that epidural anesthesia is not contraindicating in clinical practice within the interval of 80-100x$10^{-3}mm^{-3}$ (Stamer et al., 2007; Beilin et al., 1997; Van Veen et al., 2010).

Safe administration of epidural techniques to thrombocytopenic patients depends not only on the absolute platelet number but also on the reason underlying the thrombocytopenia, the rate at which the number of platelets decrease and the presence of a coagulopathy (Douglas & Ballem, 2008; Kam et al., 2004). Presence of coagulopathy contraindicates the use of regional anesthesia. However, a neuraxial block can be used in thrombocytopenic patients when their platelet quantity is adequate and stable, platelet functions are normal and there is no clinical evidence of a coagulopathy (Van Veen et al., 2010). The anesthetist should decide on a regional anesthesia on such patients after assessing the risks and benefits involved.

Since there is the risk of developing epidural hematoma in thrombocytopenic patients when either inserting or removing an epidural catheter, it is necessary to check the number of platelets before the procedure. The epidural catheter should be removed at the earliest opportunity when clinical data verifies that there is no coagulopathy involved (Douglas, 2001).

2.4 Patient refusal

A face-to-face interview should be held with the patient and the benefit-loss balance of the intended method should be explained. The procedure should not be attempted before obtaining the patient's consent.

In regional anesthesia patient cooperation is required to a certain extent. Achieving this may be difficult or even impossible in patients with dementia, psychosis or emotional dysregulation (Morgan et al., 2008).

2.5 Hemodynamic instability

The observable cardiovascular effect of an epidural anesthesia is complex and variable, and it is associated with a number of factors. The magnitude of sympathetic denervation, balance of sympathetic and parasympathetic activities, pharmacological effect of systemically absorbed local anesthetics, adrenalin content of anesthetic solutions, blood distribution associated with cardiac filling and cardiovascular functions of patients all play a role in the circulatory effect of an epidural anesthesia (Veering & Cousins, 2000).

The cardiovascular response of an epidural anesthesia depends not only on the somatic, sensory and blocked motor fibres but also on the decrease in preganglionic sympathetic tone. Local anesthetics administered to the epidural area pass into the systemic circulation by being absorbed through a local perfusion and cause a blockage of the sympathetic system (Hickey et al., 1986; Shimoji et al., 1987).

The individual cardiovascular response to the sympathetic blockage differs according to the pre-blockage degree of sympathetic tones (Veering & Cousins, 2000). Clinical use of epidural anesthesia is limited due to its risk of aggravating a preexisting systemic hypotension.

2.6 Increased intracranial pressure

Intracranial pressure (ICP) changes are characterized by the change of complains in the intracranial compartment. There is a close relationship between intracranial volume changes and ICP. When complains decrease, intracranial content increases. When ICP increases, blood flow to the brain decreases and the cerebral perfusion pressure declines (Adams & Rapper,1997).

The effect of lumbar epidural anethesia on intracranial pressure (ICP) has been studied both in animals (Bengis & Guyton, 1977)and humans (Usubiaga et al., 1967). It is known that epidural injections, at least transiently, increase ICP. With the increase in ICP, the elastance and resistance of the epidural area also increase (Grocott & Mutch, 1996). Intracranial hypertension has long been considered a contraindication to epidural anesthesia.

2.7 Local or systemic infection

The latest structural and functional studies showed that there is a firm interaction between inflammation, coagulation and fibrinolytic system (Esmon, 2003). Inflammation initiates clotting, impairs fibrinolytic system and decreases the activity of natural anticoagulant mechanisms. When inflammation starts as a local infection, coagulation activation begins as a host response to prevent propagation of microorganisms in the systemic circulation. Only in patients with very severe infection, the systemic coagulation system is activated when inflammatory cytokines disseminate in the circulation (Chrousos, 1995; Harris BH & Gelfand, 1995).

It is still controversial to use neuraxial anesthesia in patients with sepsis and systemic inflammatory response syndrome (SIRS) due to the concern that it might worsen hemodynamic instability and trigger potential problems. Active protein C therapy can be used in treating patients with serious sepsis. Insertion of an epidural catheter is contraindicated in patients with serious sepsis who are undergoing an active protein C therapy (Horlocker et al., 2003). Use of an epidural catheter in these patients will not only expose them to a higher risk but will also prevent the use of APC which would improve the patient's treatment (Gibson &Terblanche, 2011).

2.8 Pre-existing neurological diseases

It has been controversial in the past and also in our time to use neuraxial blocks in patients with a neuromuscular disease (Schmitt et al., 2004; Al-Nasser, 2002). Neuraxial blocks are hesitantly used because there is not a unique guideline for these diseases, the published data contradict each other and local anesthetics involve a potential risk of neurotoxicity (Martucci et al., 2011; Dolmass et al., 2003).

The symptoms may worsen after the block in patients who previously had a neurologic deficit or a demyelinating disease. It is impossible to differentiate whether such condition resulted from the complications developed after the block or the exacerbation of the existing disease. Some clinicians oppose, for this reason, to use neuraxial blocks in such patients (Morgan et al., 2008).

The basic problem is the lack of controlled studies to assess the potential risk that may increase in various neurologic diseases after a neuraxial application. There is also a theoretic risk of some complications (local anesthetic toxicity, nerve damage, hemorrhage and infection) which develop secondary to a regional anesthesia in this specific group of patients. However, there are a limited number of case reports showing that regional anesthesia is not accompanied by the underlying aggravation (Pogson et al., 2000; Stoelting & Dierdorf, 2002).

A neuraxial blockage may be preferred after a detailed discussion of the individual disease is made without overlooking the risk of worsening the neurologic function.

3. Conclusion

Anesthesia societies, in patient with coagulation defect and anticoagulant agents uses, developed guidelines to help anesthesiologists to predict the optimal time for neuraxial techniques. These guidelines based on clinical experinces and case series. The most basic common features of these guidelines are the nontraumatic implementation of the neuraxial analgesia by experienced anesthesiologists. Of course the management of individual risks and benefits must perform carefully.

4. References

Abramovitz, S.&Beilin, S. (2003). Thrombocytopenia, low molecular weight heparin, and obstetric anesthesia. Anesthesiology Clinics of North America, 21,1, pp. 99-109

Adams, G. L., Manson, R. J., Turner, I., Sindram, D.& Lawson, J. H. (2007). The balance of thrombosis and hemorrhage in surgery. Hematology/ Oncology Clinics of North America, 21,1, pp. 13-24

Adams, R.A. & Rapper, A.H. (1997). *Principles of Neurology*, 6th Edition, McGrow Hill, New York

Aiach, M., Borgel, D., Gaussem, P., Emmerich, J., Alhenc-Gelas, M. & Gandrille, S. (1997). Protein C and protein S deficiencies.Seminars in Hematology, 34, pp. 205–17

Al-Nasser, B. (2002). Local toxicity of local anesthetics do experimental data apply to clinical manifestations? Anesthesia, 57, 12, pp. 1236-37

Ansell, J., Hirsh, J., Poller, L., Bussey, H., Jacobson, A. & Hylek, E. (2004). The pharmacology and management of the vitamin k antagonists. Chest, 126, pp. 204S–233S

Armand, R. & Hess, J.R. (2003). Treating coagulopathy in trauma patients. Transfusion Medicine Reviews, 17, 3, pp. 223-31

Asselta, R., Tenchini, M.L. & Duga, S. (2006). Inherited defects of coagulation factor V: the hemorrhagic side. Journal of Thrombosis and Haemostasis, 4, pp. 26–34

Begbie, M.E., Wallace, G.M. & Shovlin, C.L. (2003). Hereditary haemorrhagic telangiectasia (Osler-Weber-Rendu syndrome): a view from the 21st century. Postgraduate Medical Journal, 79, pp. 18–24

Beilin, Y., Zahn, J. & Comerford, M. (1997). Safe epidural analgesia in thirty parturients with platelet counts between 69,000 and 98,000 mm(-3). Anesthesia Analgesia, 85, 2, pp. 85-8

Belgian Guidelines. (2000). Belgian Guidelines concerning drug induced alterations of coagulation and central neuraxial anesthesia. Acta Anaesthesiologica Belgica, 51, pp. 101–04

Bengis, R.G. & Guyton, A.C. (1977). Some pressure and fluid dynamic characteristics of the canine epidural space. The American Journal of Physiology, 232, 3, pp. H255-9

Bergqvist, D., Lindblad, B. & Mätzsch, T. (1993). Risk of combining low molecular weight heparin for thromboprophylaxis and epidural or spinal anesthesia. Seminars in Thrombosis and Hemostasis, 19 (Suppl 1), pp. 147–51

Bernhardt, A., Bald, C., Helfrich, U. & Haubelt, H. (2008). Continuous lumbar epidural anesthesia: insertion a patient with unrecognized classical hemophilia A. Anaesthesist, 57, pp. 578–81

Bernard, J. (1983). History of congenital hemorrhagic thrombocytopathic dystrophy. Blood Cells, 9, pp. 179 -93

Birnbach, D.J. & Grunebaum, A. (1991). The anticoagulated parturient. In: Anesthetic and Obstetric Management of High Risk Pregnancy, Datta S (Ed.), pp. 522-35, St. Louis: Mosby Year Book. The

Boehringer-Ingelheim.(2009). Pradaxa - Summary of product characteristics, 22-03-2009, Available from http://www.emea.europa.eu/humandocs/PDFs/EPAR/pradaxa/H-829-PI-en.pdf

Boneu, B., Necciari, J., Cariou, R., Sié, P., Gabaig, A.M., Kieffer, G., Dickinson, J., Lamond, G., Moelker, H. & Mant, T. (1995). Pharmacokinetics and tolerance of the natural pentasaccharide (SR90107/Org31540) with high affinity to antithrombin III in man. Thrombosis and Haemostasis, 74, 6, pp. 1468–473

British Committee for Standards in Haematology General Haematology Task Force, (2003). Guidelines for the investigation and management of idiopathic thrombocytopenic purpura in adults, children and in pregnancy. British Journal of Haematology, 120, pp. 574–596

Bromage, P.R. (1993). Neurologic complications of regional anesthesia for obstetrics. In: Anesthesia for obstetrics, Shnider SM, Levinson G, eds, pp. 443-4, 3rd ed. Baltimore: Williams & Wilkins

Burger, W., Chemnitius, J.M., Kneissl, G.D. & Rücker, G. (2005). Low-dose aspirin for secondary cardiovascular prevention - cardiovascular risks after its perioperative withdrawal versus bleeding risks with its continuation- review. Journal of Internal Medicine , 257, pp. 399–414

Cahill, M.R. & Colvin, B.T. (1997). Haemophilia. Postgraduate Medical Journal, 73, 858, pp. 201-6

Caliezi, C., Tsakiris, D.A., Behringer, H., Kühne, T. & Marbet, G.A. (1998). Two consecutive pregnancies and deliveries in a patient with von Willebrand's disease type 3. Haemophilia, 4, pp. 845-849

Cerneca, F., Ricci, G., Simeone, R., Malisano, M., Alberico, S. & Guaschino, S. (1997). Coagulation and fibrinolysis changes in normal pregnancy. Increased levels of procoagulants and reduced levels of inhibitors during pregnancy induce a hypercoagulable state, combined with a reactive fibrinolysis. European Journal of Obstetrics, Gynecology, and Reproductive Biology, 73, pp. 31–36

Chesebro, B. B., Rahn, P., Carles, M., Esmon, CT., Xu, J., Brohi, K., Frith, D., Pittet, J.F. & Cohen, M.J. (2009). Increase in activated proteinCmediates acute traumatic coagulopathy. Shock, 32, pp. 659–65

Chow, L., Farber, M.K. & Camann, W.R. (2011). Anesthesia in the pregnant patient with hematologic disorders. Hematology/Oncology Clinics of North America, 25, 2, pp. 425-43

Chrousos, G.P. (1995). The hypothalamic-pituitary-adrenal axis and immune-mediated inflammation. New England Journal of Medicine, 332, pp. 1351–62

Cohen, S., Daitch, J.S., Amar, D. & Goldiner, P.L. (1989). Epidural analgesia for labor and delivery in a patient with von Willebrand's disease. Regional Anesthesia, 14, pp. 95-97

CLASP (Collaborative Low-dose Aspirin Study in Pregnancy) Collaborative Group. (1994). CLASP: a randomised trial of low-dose aspirin for the prevention and treatment of pre-eclampsia among 9364 pregnant women. Lancet, 343, pp. 619–29

Colman, R.W., Clowes, A.W. & George, J.N. (2001). Overview of hemostasis. In: Hemostasis and thrombosis: Basic principles and clinical practice. Colman RW, Hirsh J, Marder VJ, et al, eds. Philadelphia: Lippincott, Williams & Wilkins

Dalmas, A.F., Texier, C., Ducloy Bouthors, A.S. & Krivosic Horber, R. (2003). Obstetrical analgesia and anesthesia in multiple sclerosis. Annales Francaises Anesthesia Reanimation, 22, 10, pp. 861-4

Dasgupta, H., Blankenship, J.C., Wood, G.C., Frey, C.M., Demko, S.L. & Menapace, F.J. (2000). Thrombocytopenia complicating treatment with intravenous glycoprotein IIb/ IIIa receptor inhibitors: a pooled analysis. American Heart Journal, 140, 2, pp. 206–11

Dhar, P., Abramovitz, S., DiMichele, D., Gibb, C.B. & Gadalla, F. (2003). Management of pregnancy in a patient with severe haemophilia A. British Journal of Anesthesia, 91, pp. 432–35

DiMichele, D.& Neufeld, E.J. (1998). Hemophilia. A new approach to an old disease. Hematology/ Oncology Clinics of North America, 12, pp. 1315-44

Donegan, E., Stratmann, G. &Kan, T.N.(2007). Hemostasis. In: Basics of Anesthesia. 5th ed., R.K. Stoelting, R.D. Miller, (Ed.), 331-46, Philadelphia, Churchill Livingstone

Douglas, M. J. (2001) . Platelets, the parturient and regional anesthesia. International Journal of Obstetric Anesthesia, 10, 2, pp. 113–20

Douglas, M.& Ballem, P. (2008). Blood disorders. In: Obstetric Anesthesia and Uncommon Disorders (ed. by D. Gambling, M. Douglas & R. McKay), pp. 303–320, 2nd edn. Cambridge University Press, New York.

Dunn, A.& Turpie, A.G.G. (2003). Perioperative management of patients on oral anticoagulants: a systematic review. Archives of Internal Medicine, 163, pp. 901–08

Esmon, C.T. (1989). The roles of protein C and thrombomodulin in the regulation of blood coagulation. The Journal of Biology Chemistry, 264, pp. 4743–6

Esmon, C.T. (2003). Inflammation and thrombosis. Journal of Thrombosis and Haemostasis, 1, pp. 1343–48

Faillace, W.J., Warrier, I. & Canady, A.I. (1989). Paraplegia after lumbar puncture. In an infant with previously undiagnosed hemophilia A. Treatment and peri-operative considerations. Clinical Pediatrics, 28, pp. 136–8

Falati, S., Gross, P., Merrill-Skoloff, G., Furie, B.C.& Furie, B. (2002). Real-time in vivo imaging of platelets, tissue factor and fibrin during arterial thrombus formation in the mouse.Nature Medicine, 8, 10, pp. 1175-81. Epub 2002 Sep 16

Fogerty, A.E. & Connors, J.M. (2009). Management of inherited thrombophilia in pregnancy. Current Opinion in Endocrinology, Diabetes, and Obesity, 16,6, pp. 464-9

Gailani, D.& Broze, G. J. Jr. (1991). Factor XI activation in a revised model of blood coagulation. Science, 253, 5022, pp. 909-12

Gando, S.(2001). Disseminated intravascular coagulation in trauma patients. Seminars in Thrombosis and Haemostasis, 27, pp. 585–91

Gando, S., Tedo, I., Hanaoka, Y., Makise, N., Tsujinaga, H. & Kubota, M. (1988). Blood coagulation and fibrinolysis in anesthesia and operations, with special reference to FPA, FPB beta 15-42. Masui, 37, 4, pp.451-6

Gando, S., Tedo, I. & Kubota, M.(1992). Posttrauma coagulation and fibrinolysis. Critical Care Medicine, 20, pp. 594–600

George, J.N., Caen, J.P. & Nurden, A.T. (1990). Glanzmann's thrombasthenia: the spectrum of clinical disease. Blood, 75, 7, pp. 1383-95

Gibson, B. & Terblanche, C. (2011). Anaesthetic management of patients with severe sepsis. British Journal of Anesthesia, 106, 3, pp. 416-7; author reply 417

Gogarten, W. (2006). The influence of new antithrombotic drugs on regional anesthesia. Current Opinion in Anaesthesiology, 19, pp. 545–50

Gogarten, W., Van Aken, H., Wulf, H., Klose, R., Vandermeulen, E. & Harenberg, J. (1997). Regional anesthesia and thromboembolism prophylaxis/anticoagulation. Anesthesiology and Intensive Care Medicine, 38, pp. 623–28

Gogarten, W., Vandermeulen, E., Van Aken, H., Kozek, S., Llau, J.V. & Samama, C.M. (2010). Regional anesthesia and antithrombotic agents: recommendations of the European Society of Anaesthesioogy. European Journal of Anaesthesiology, 27, pp. 999–1015

Greer, I.A., Lowe, G.D., Walker, J.J. & Forbes, C.D. (1991). Haemorrhagic problems in obstetrics and gynaecology in patients with congenital coagulopathies. British Journal of Obstetrics and Gynaecology, 98, pp. 909-918

Greinacher, A. (2004). Lepirudin: a bivalent direct thrombin inhibitor for anticoagulation therapy. Expert Review of Cardiovascular Therapy, 2, 3, pp. 339–57

Grocott, H.P. & Mutch, W.A. (1996). Epidural anesthesia and acutely increased intracranial pressure. Lumbar epidural space hydrodynamics in a porcine model. Anesthesiology, 85, 5, pp. 1086-91

Guffey, P.J. & McKay, W.R.(2010). Case report: epidural hematoma nine days after removal of a labor epidural catheter. Anesthesia and Analgesia, 111, 4, pp. 992-5. Epub 2010 Jul 30

Han, I.S., Chung, E.Y. & Hahn, Y.J. (2010). Spinal epidural hematoma after epidural anesthesia in a patient receiving enoxaparin -A case report- Korean Journal of Anesthesiology, 59, 2, pp. 119-22. Epub 2010 Aug 20

Hara, K., Kishi, N. & Sata, T. (2009). Considerations for epidural anesthesia in a patient with type 1 von Willebrand disease. Journal of Anesthesia, 23, 4, pp. 597-600. Epub 2009 Nov 18

Harker, L.A. & Slichter, S.J. (1972). The bleeding time as a screening test for evaluation of platelet function. The New England Journal of Medicine, 287, 4, pp. 155-9

Harris, B.H. & Gelfand, J.A. (1995). The immune response to trauma. Seminars in Pediatric Surgery, 4, pp. 77–82

Hess, J.R. & Lawson, J.H. (2006) . The coagulapaty of trauma versus disseminated intravascular coagulation. Journal of Trauma, 60, 6 Suppl, pp. S12-9

Hereditary Hemorrhagic Telangiectasia Foundation International Inc. Hereditary Hemorrhagic Telangiectasia Summary for Physicians and Health Care Providers, hctpV/www.hht.org/content/hht-summary. html. Accessed May 11, 2007

Hickey, R., Albin, M.S., Bunegin, L. & Gelineau, J. (1986). Autoregulation of spinal cord blood flow: is the cord a microcosm of the brain?.Stroke, 17, 6, pp. 1183-9

Hirsh, J.& Raschke, R. (2004). Heparin and low molecular-weight heparin. Chest, 126, pp. 188S–203S

Hirsh, J., Warkentin, T.E., Shaughnessy, S.G., Anand, S.S., Halperin, J.L., Raschke, R., Granger, C., Ohman, E.M. & Dalen, J.E. (2001). Heparin and low-molecular-weight heparin: mechanisms of action, pharmacokinetics, dosing, monitoring, efficacy, and safety. Chest, 119(Suppl), pp. 64S–94S

Hoffman, M.& Monroe, D.M. 3rd. (2001). A cell-based model of hemostasis. Thrombosis and Haemostasis, 85, pp. 958-65

Hoffman, M.& Monroe, D. M. (2007).Coagulation 2006: a modern view of hemostasis. Hematology/ Oncology Clinics of North America, 21, 1, pp. 1-11

Horlocker, T.T., Bajwa, Z.H., Ashraf, Z., Khan, S., Wilson, J.L., Sami, N., Peeters-Asdourian, C., Powers, C.A., Schroeder, D.R., Decker, P.A. & Warfield, C.A. (2002). Risk assessment of hemorrhagic complications associated with nonsteroidal antiinflammatory medications in ambulatory pain clinic patients undergoing epidural steroid injection. Anesthesia and Analgesia, 95, pp. 1691–97

Horlocker, T.T., Wedel, D.J., Schroeder, D.R., Rose, S.H., Elliott, B.A., McGregor, D.G. &Wong, G.Y. (1995). Preoperative antiplatelet therapy does not increase the risk of spinal hematoma associated with regional anesthesia. Anesthesia and Analgesia, 80, pp. 303–09

Horlocker, T.T. & Wedel, D.J. (1998). Anticoagulation and neuraxial block: historical perspective, anesthetic implications, and risk management. Regional Anesthesia Pain Medicine, 23, pp. 129–34

Horlocker, T.T., Wedel, D.J., Benzon, H., Brown, D.L., Enneking, F.K., Heit, J.A., Mulroy, M.F., Rosenquist, R.W., Rowlingson, J., Tryba, M. & Yuan, C.S. (2003). Regional anesthesia in the anticoagulated patient: Defining the risks (The Second ASRA Consensus Conference on Neuraxial Anesthesia and Anticoagulation). Regional Anesthesia Pain Medicine, 28, pp. 172–97

Hornyak, T.J. & Shafer, J. A. (1992). Interactions of factor XIII with fibrin as substrate and cofactor. Biochemistry, 31, 2, pp. 423-9

Huang, F. & Hong, E. (2004). Platelet glycoprotein IIb/IIIa inhibition and its clinical use. Current Medicinal Chemistry. Cardiovascular and Hematological Agents, 2, 3, pp. 187–96

Hull, R.D., Pineo, G.F. & MacIsaac, S. (2000). Low-molecular-weight heparin prophylaxis: preoperative versus postoperative initiation in patients undergoing elective hip surgery. Thrombosis Research, 101, V155–V162

Ibbotson, T. & Perry, C.M., Ibbotson, T. & Perry, CM. (2002). Danaparoid: a review of its use in thromboembolic and coagulation disorders. Drugs, 62, 15, pp. 2283–314

Jones, B.P., Bell, E.A. & Maroof, M. (1999). Epidural labor analgesia in a parturient with von Willebrand's disease type IIA and severe preeclampsia. Anesthesiology , 90, pp. 1219-1220

Kam, P.C., Thompson, S.A. & Liew, A.C. (2004). Thrombocytopenia in the parturient. Anesthesia, 59, 3, pp. 255-64

Kadir, R., Chi, C. & Bolton-Maggs, P. (2009). Pregnancy and rare bleeding disorders. Haemophilia, 15, pp. 990–1005

Kadir, R.A., Lee, C.A., Sabin, C.A., Pollard, D. & Economides, D.L. (1998). Pregnancy in women with von Willebrand's disease or factor XI deficiency. British Journal of Obstetrics and Gynaecology, 105, pp. 314-321

Kathiresan, S., Shiomura, J. & Jang, I.K. (2002). Argatroban. Journal of Thrombosis and Thrombolysis, 13, 1, 41–47

Kaplan, K.L.(2003). Direct thrombin inhibitors. Expert Opinion on Pharmacotherapy, 4, 5, pp. 653–66

Kessler, I., Lancet, M., Borenstein, R., Berrebi, A. & Mogilner, B.M. (1982). The obstetrical management of patients with immunologic thrombocytopenic purpura. International Journal of Gynaecologl Obstetrics , 20, pp. 23–8.

Kostopanagiotou, G., Siafaka, I., Sikiotis, C. & Smyrniotis, V. (2004). Anesthetic and perioperative management of a patient with Bernard-Soulier syndrome. Journal of Clinical Anesthesia, 16, 6, pp. 458-60

Kövesi, T. & Royston, D. (2002). Is there a bleeding problem with platelet-active drugs? British Journal of Anesthesia, 88, pp. 159–62

Kubitza, D., Becka ,M., Wensing, G., Voith, B. & Zuehlsdorf, M. (2005). Safety, pharmacodynamics, and pharmacokinetics of BAY 59–7939–an oral, direct Factor

Xa inhibitor–after multiple dosing in healthy male subjects. European Journal of Clinical Pharmacology, 61, 12, pp. 873–80

Le Gouez, A., Roger-Christoph, S., Abbes, M. & Benhamou, D. (2011). Anesthetic management of parturients with defects in coagulation factor V. International Journal of Obstetrics Anesthesia, 20, 1, pp. 97-8. Epub 2010 Oct 29

Lee, C.A., Chi, C., Pavord, S.R., Bolton-Maggs, P.H., Pollard, D., Hinchcliffe-Wood, A. & Kadir, R.A. (2006). The obstetric and gynaecological management of women with inherited bleeding disorders--review with guidelines produced by a taskforce of UK Haemophilia Centre Doctors' Organization. Haemophilia, 12, 4, pp. 301-36

Levi, M. & Ten Cate, H. (1993). Disseminated intravascular coagulation. The New England Journal of Medicine, 341, pp. 586 -92

Levy, J.H., Dutton, R.P., Hemphill, J.C. 3rd., Shander, A., Cooper, D., Paidas, M.J., Kessler, C.M., Holcomb, J.B. & Lawson, J.H. (2010). Multidisciplinary Approach to the Challenge of Hemostasis. Anesthesia and Analgesia, 110, 2, pp. 354-64. Epub 2009 Dec 10

Levy, J.H., Tanaka, K.A. & Dietrich, W. (2008). Perioperative hemostatic management of patients treated with vitamin K antagonists. Anesthesiology, 109, 5, pp. 918-26

Li, S.L., Wang, D.X. & Ma, D. (2010). Epidural hematoma after neuraxial blockade: a retrospective report from China. Anesthesia and Analgesia, 111, 5, pp. 1322-4. Epub 2010 Aug 12

Litz, R.J., Gottschlich, B. & Stehr, S.N. (2004). Spinal epidural hematoma after spinal anesthesia in a patient treated with clopidogrel and enoxaparin. Anesthesiology, 101, pp. 1467–70

Llau, J.V., De Andrés, J., Gomar, C., Gómez, A., Hidalgo, F., Sahagún, J. & Torres, L.M. (2001). Drugs that alter hemostasis and regional anesthetic techniques: safety guidelines. Consensus conference (Spanish). Revista Espanola Anestesiologica Reanimacion, 48, pp. 270–78

Llau, J.V., De Andrés , J., Gomar , C., Gómez , Z., Hidalgo, F. & Torres , L.M. (2005). Guidelines of hemostasis inhibiting drugs and neuraxial anesthesia (Spanish). Revista Espanola Anestesiologica Reanimacion, 52, pp. 413–20

Llau, , J.V., De Andrés, J., Gomar, C., Gómez, Z., Hidalgo, F. & Torres, L.M. (2005). Hemostasis-altering drugs and techniques for regional anesthesia and analgesia: safety recommendations (Spanish). Rev Esp Anestesiol Reanim , 52, pp. 248–250

Llau, J.V., De Andrés, J., Gomar, C., Gómez-Luque, A., Hidalgo, F. & Torres, L.M. (2007). Anticlotting drugs and regional anaesthetic and analgesic techniques: comparative update of the safety recommendations. European Journal of Anaesthesiology, 24, 5, pp. 387-98. Epub 2007 Jan 8

Lomax, S. & Edgcombe, H. (2009). Anesthetic implications for the parturient with hereditary hemorrhagic telangiectasia. Canadian Journal of Anesthesia, 56, 5, pp. 374-84. Epub 2009 Mar 28

Lubenow, N.& Greinacher, A.(2002). Hirudin in heparin-induced thrombocytopenia. Seminars in Thrombosis and Hemostasis, 28, 5, pp. 431–38

Maclean, P.S. & Tait, R.C. (2007). Hereditary and acquired antithrombin deficiency: epidemiology, pathogenesis and treatment options. Drugs, 67, 10, pp. 1429-40

Mannucci, P.M. & Tuddenham, E.G. (2001). The hemophilias--from royal genes to gene therapy. The New England Journal of Medicine, 344, 23, pp. 1773-9
Martini, W.Z.(2009). Coagulopathy by hypothermia and acidosis: mechanisms of thrombin generation and fibrinogen availability. Journal of Trauma, 67, pp. 202–09
Martucci, G., Di Lorenzo, A., Polito, F. & Acampa, L. (2011). A 12-month follow-up for neurological complication after subarachnoid anesthesia in a parturient affected by multiple sclerosis. European Review for Medical Pharmacological Sciences, 15, 4, pp. 458-60
McQuaid, K.R. & Laine, L. (2006). Systematic review and meta-analysis of adverse events of low-dose aspirin and clopidogrel in randomized controlled trials. The American Journal of Medicine, 119, pp. 624–38
Mentegazzi, F., Danelli, G., Ghisi, D., Tosi, M., Gennari, A. & Fanelli, G. (2005). Locoregional anesthesia and coagulation. Minerva Anestesiologica, 71:, pp. 497–499
Milaskiewicz, R.M., Holdcroft, A. & Letsky, E. (1990). Epidural anesthesia and von Willebrand's disease. Anesthesia , 45, pp. 462-464
Moen, V., Dahlgren, N. & Irestedt, L. (2004). Severe neurological complications after central neuraxial blockades in Sweden 1990-1999. Anesthesiology, 101, pp. 950-9
Monroe, D. M., Roberts, H. R.& Hoffman, M. (1994). Platelet procoagulant complex assembly in a tissue factor-initiated system.British Journal of Haematology, 88, 2, pp. 364-71
Morgan, G.E., Mikhail, M.S. & Murray, M.J. (2008). Spinal, epidural and caudal blocks. In: Clinical Anesthesiology, pp. 298-310, 4th Ed. Appleton & Lange, Stamford
Ordog, G.J., Wasserberger, J. & Balasubramanium, S. (1985). Coagulation abnormalities in traumatic shock. Annals of Emergency Medicine, 14, pp. 650–55
Pamnani, A., Rosenstein, M., Darwich, A. & Wolfson, A. (2010). Neuraxial anesthesia for labor and cesarean delivery in a parturient with hereditary antithrombin deficiency on recombinant human antithrombin infusion therapy. Journal of Clinical Anesthesia, 22, 6, pp. 450-3
Patrono, C., Coller, B., FitzGerald, G.A., Hirsh, J. & Roth, G. (2004). Platelet active drugs: the relationships among dose, effectiveness, and side effects. Chest, 126, pp. 234S–64S
Punnonen, R., Nyman, D., Grönroos, M. & Wallén, O. (1981). Von Willebrand's disease and pregnancy. Acta Obstetricia et Gynecologica Scandinavica, 60, pp. 507-09
Rasmus, K.T., Rottman, R.L., Kotelko, D.M., Wright, W.C., Stone, J.J. & Rosenblatt, R.M. (1989). Unrecognized thrombocytopenia and regional anesthesia in parturients: a retrospective review. Obstetrics and Gynecology, 73, pp. 943- 6
Reitsma, P.H. (1997). Protein C deficiency: from gene defects to disease. Thrombosis and Haemostasis, 78, pp. 344–50
Robson, R., White, H., Aylward, P. & Frampton, C. (2002). Bivalirudin pharmacokinetics and pharmacodynamics: effect of renal function, dose, and gender. Clinical Pharmacology and Therapeutics, 71, 6, pp. 433–39
Rodeghiero, F., Castaman, G. & Dini, E. (1987). Epidemiological investigation of the prevalence of von Willebrand's disease. Blood, 69, pp. 454-459
Rolbin, S.H., Abbott, D., Musclow, E., Papsin, F., Lie, L.M. & Freedman, J.(1988). Epidural anesthesia in pregnant patients with low platelet counts. Obstetrics and Gynecology, 71, pp. 918- 20

Rosenberg, R.D. (1975). Actions and interactions of antithrombin III and heparin. The New England Journal of Medicine, 292, pp. 146-51

Samama, C.M., Bastien, O., Forestier, F., Denninger, M.H., Isetta, C., Juliard, J.M., Lasne, D., Leys, D. & Mismetti, P. (2002). Antiplatelet agents in the perioperative period: expert recommendations of the French Society of Anesthesiology and Intensive Care (SFAR) 2001 - Summary statement. Canadian Journal of Anesthesia, 49, pp. S26-S35

Sawamura, A., Hayakawa, M., Gando, S., Kubota, N., Sugano, M., Wada, T. & Katabami, K. (2009). Disseminated intravascular coagulation with a fibrinolytic phenotype at an early phase of trauma predicts mortality. Thrombosis Research, 124, pp. 608–13

Schmitt, H.J., Muenster, T. & Schmitt, J. (2004). Central neural blockade in Charcot- Marie-Tooth disease. Canadian Journal of Anesthesia, 51, 10, pp. 1049-50

Serebruany, V.L., Steinhubl, S.R., Berger, P.B., Malinin, A.I., Baggish, J.S., Bhatt, D.L. & Topol, E.J. (2005). Analysis of risk of bleeding complications after different doses of aspirin in 192 036 patients enrolled in 31 randomized controlled trials. The American Journal of Cardiology, 95, pp. 1218–22

Shimoji, K., Sato, Y., Endoh, H., Taga, K., Fujiwara, N. & Fukuda, S. (1987). Relation between spinal cord and epidural blood flow. Stroke, 18, 6, pp. 1128-32

Silverman, R., Kwiatkowski, T., Bernstein, S., Sanders, N., Hilgartner, M., Cahill-Bordas, M., Jackson, K. & Lipton, R. (1993). Safety of lumbar puncture in patients with hemophilia. Annals of Emergency Medicine, 22, pp. 1739–42

Stamer, U.M., Stuber, F., Wiese, R., Wulf, H. & Meuser, T. (2007). Contraindications to regional anesthesia in obstetrics: a survey of German practice. International Journal of Obstetric Anesthesia, 16, pp. 328–335

Sternberg, T.L., Bailey, M.K., Lazarchick, J. & Brahen, N.H. (1991). Protein C deficiency as a cause of pulmonary embolismin the perioperative period. Anesthesiology, 74, pp. 364–6

Stoelting, R.K.& Dierdorf, S.F. (2002). Anesthesia and Co-Existing Disease. 4th ed. Philadelphia, PA: Churchill Livingstone

Tanaka, K.A., Key, N. S. & Levy, J. H. (2009). Blood coagulation: hemostasis and thrombin regulation. Anesthesia and Analgesia, 108, pp. 1433-46

Tiede, A., Tait, R.C., Shaffer, D.W., Baudo, F., Boneu, B., Dempfle, C.E., Horellou, M.H., Klamroth, R., Lazarchick, J., Mumford, A.D., Schulman, S., Shiach, C., Bonfiglio, L.J., Frieling, J.T., Conard, J. & von Depka, M. (2008). Antithrombin alfa in hereditary antithrombin deficient patients: a phase 3 study of prophylactic intravenous administration in high risk situations. Thrombosis and Haemostasis, 99, pp. 616-22

Tripodi, A., Chantarangkul, V., Primignani, M., Fabris, F., Dell'Era, A., Sei, C. & Mannucci, P.M. (2007). The international normalized ratio calibrated for cirrhosis (INR(liver)) normalizes prothrombin time results for model for end-stage liver disease calculation. Hepatology, 46, 2, pp. 520-7

Tuddenham, E.G.D.& Cooper, D.N. (1994). The molecular genetics of haemostasis and its inherited disorders. Oxford monographs in medical genetics no. 25. Oxford, England: Oxford University Press

Tufano, A., Cerbone, A.M. & Di Minno, G. (2002). The use of antithrombotic drugs in older people. Minerva Medica, 93, pp. 13–26

Turpini, R. & Stefanini, M. (1959). The nature and mechanism of the hemostatic breakdown in the course of experimental hemorrhagic shock. Journal of Clinical Investigation, 38, pp. 53–65

Tyagi, A.& Bhattacharya, A. (2002). Central neuraxial blocks and anticoagulation: a review of current trends. European Journal of Anaesthesiology, 19, pp. 317–329

Usubiaga, J.E., Usubiaga, L.E., Brea, L.M. & Goyena, R. (1967). Effect of saline injections on epidural and subarachnoid space pressures and relation to postspinal anesthesia headache. *Anesthesia and Analgesia*, 46, 3, pp. 293-6

Vandermeulen, E.P., Van Aken, H. & Vermylen, J. (1994). Anticoagulants and spinal epidural anesthesia. Anesthesia and Analgesia, 79, pp. 1165–17

Vandermeulen, E., Singelyn, F., Vercauteren, M., Brichant, J.F., Ickx, B.E. & Gautier, P. (2005). Belgian guidelines concerning central neural blockade in patients with drug induced alteration of coagulation: an update. Acta Anaesthesiologica Belgica, 56, pp. 139–46

Vandermeulen, E. (2010). Regional anesthesia and anticoagulation. Best Practice &Research. Clinical Anaesthesiology, 24, 1, pp. 121-31

van Veen, J.J., Nokes, T.J. & Makris, M. (2010). The risk of spinal haematoma following neuraxial anesthesia or lumbar puncture in thrombocytopenic individuals. British Journal of Haematology, 148, 1, pp. 15-25. Epub 2009 Sep 22

Varughese, J. & Cohen, A.J. (2007). Experience with epidural anesthesia in pregnant women with von Willebrand disease. Haemophilia, 13, 6, pp. 730-3

Veering, B.T.& Cousins, M.J. (2000). Cardiovascular and pulmonary effects of epidural anesthesia. Anesthesia and Intensive Care, 28, 6, pp. 620-35

Vellinga, S., Steel, E., Vangenechten, I. & Gadisseur, A. (2006). Successful pregnancy in a patient with factor V deficiency: case report and review of the literature. Thrombosis and Haemostasis, 95, pp. 896–897

Walker, I.D. (1997). Congenital thrombophilia. Baillieres Clinics Obstetrics and Gynaecology, 11, pp. 431–45

Warkentin, T.E., Levine, M.N., Hirsh, J., Horsewood, P., Roberts, R.S., Gent, M. & Kelton, J.G. (1995). Heparin-induced thrombocytopenia in patients treated with low-molecular-weight heparin or unfractionated heparin. New England Journal of Medicine, 332, pp. 1330–335

Webert, K.E., Mittal, R., Sigouin, C., Heddle, N.M. & Kelton, J.G. (2003). A retrospective 11-year analysis of obstetric patients with idiopathic thrombocytopenic purpura. Blood, 102, 13, pp. 4306-11

Weitz, J.I. (1997). Low-molecular-weight heparins. New England Journal of Medicine, 337, pp. 688–98

Weitz, J.I., Hirsh, J. & Samama, M.M. (2004). New anticoagulant drugs. Chest, 126, pp. 265S–286S

Weitz, J.I., Hirsh, J. & Samama, M.M. (2008). Physicians ACoC. New antithrombotic drugs: American College of Chest Physicians Evidence-Based Clinical Practice Guidelines (8th Edition). Chest, 133, pp. 234S– 56S

Wilde, M.I. & Markham A. (1997). Danaparoid. A review of its pharmacology and clinical use in the management of heparininduced thrombocytopenia. Drugs, 54, 6, pp. 903-24

Wolberg, A.S., Meng, Z.H., Monroe, D. M. 3rd. & Hoffman, M. (2004). A systemic evaluation of the effect of temperature on coagulation enzyme activity and platelet function. Journal of Trauma, 56, pp. 1221-28

Yeh, R.W.& Jang, I.K. (2006). Argatroban: update. American Heart Journal, 151, pp. 1131-138